SCIENTIFIC CHIROPRACTIC

Paul Smallie, DC, HHD

Library of Congress Catalog Number

84 62211

ISBN 0 9614296-3 1

Published in 1984 by World-Wide Books
2027 Grand Canal Boulevard 20 Stockton, CA 95207

CONTENTS

ACKNOWLEDGEMENT

Ernest G Napolitano, DC, President of New York Chiropractic College, is sincerely acknowledged for contributing a most appreciated source of inspiration and guidance in preparing this text.

-**Paul Smallie, DC**

In the broadest sense, all healing arts are based on the study of man, how he is constructed, how he functions and how he acts and reacts to his environment, to his fellowman and to his inner stresses.

-Mortimer Levine, DC

INTRODUCTION

It seems imperative that this new text be put into print to further affirm the evident fact that chiropractic as a profession is indeed scientific.

The ARCHIVES of LITERATURE RELATIVE to the SCIENCE OF CHIROPRACTIC, edited and published by the Canadian Memorial Chiropractic College, opens with this assertion:

"The dissemination of information contained in this book is long overdue... Had this book been published forty or fifty years earlier, the term -unscientific cult- would never have been levelled against chiropractic."

The editors add: "We are entering a new era in chiropractic, a scientific era ushered in by the work of chiropractors, osteopaths, medical doctors and scientists. Many researchers in these are working in parallel fields and are not aware that the product of their research is supportive to the chiropractic science. The accumulated evidence in this volume will bear tangible evidence to this fact. ...it shows chiropractic to have a sturdy foundation in scientific thought."

In the European Chiropractors Union Bulletin, 1981, volume 29, number 2, Olgierd Minkiewicz, DC, concludes an article on "A Scientific Basis For Chiropractic" with these words:

"There is great need to disprove the words 'non-scientific chiropractor' and to enter into a new scientific phase of our profession. To do so we must most definitely review the orthodox concept of the autonomic nervous system. We must realize that any new approach necessitates the discarding of many old ideas and there is usually great resistance to this, but if we wish to establish a truly scientific chiropractic, then we have no option."

Chapter I

SCIENCE

Definition

The March, 1984 issue of **WORLD-WIDE REPORT** carried a news item of highly significant information. It announced a new-found uniformity and accord for a chiropractic educational system that had very much needed just such uniformity.

The announcement needs to be communicated at the outset of this text on Scientific Chiropractic because of the importance of establishing an agreement within these united areas of chiropractic education, demonstrating the advancements in what has been agreed upon and establishing this as an official profession-initiated and profession-supported definition that now further stabilizes the profession with a dependable guideline. Mainly, it is an important documentation intended to guide, rather than to limit.

It is important because we now have an historical document representative of the combined agreement of those responsible for formulating guidelines as they apply to the educational process involved in the preparation of students for their degree of Doctor of Chiropractic.

Here was the announcement:

"Upon an historic occasion, during the Annual Meeting of January 28 and 29, 1984, in Reno, Nevada, the Board of Directors of the Council on Chiropractic Education unanimously approved and endorsed the following definition of chiropractic science:

Chiropractic is the science which concerns itself with the relationship between structure, primarily the spine, and function, primarily the nervous system of the human body as the relationship may affect the restoration and preservation of health.

1

"The definition was also unanimously approved and endorsed by the fifteen chiropractic colleges in the United States and Canada on January 26, 1984, during the Annual Meeting of the college presidents.

"During an interview with Dr Marino R Passero, the newly elected President of the Council on Chiropractic Education, he stated that the action of the CCE Board of Directors and the college presidents is another milestone for the profession. He further indicated the definition of chiropractic science shall help to establish a stronger basis for the future of chiropractic research, education and meet the health needs of the public."

This was a most welcome gift to the profession because of the now-coordinated influence it will have upon the future of chiropractic education and practice.

Chiropractic as a Science

In an abstract that appeared in the June, 1984 issue of the JOURNAL of MANIPULATIVE and PHYSIOLOGICAL THERAPEUTICS, in connection with an article -Educational Preparation for Chiropractic Clinical Research, by Jennifer R Jamison, M Ed-, it was observed that "Chiropractic is severely criticized by organized medicine for its lack of scientific proof and publications."

The medical profession has attempted to designate itself as supreme in all matters pertaining to health and presents the argument that if another profession does not subscribe to the concepts of medical science then it cannot be classified as a science. It is the contention of chiropractic science, however, that its science is separate and distinct and not dependent upon medical science for its conclusions. Medicine, as a profession, has no sole claim to biological science. It is available to all. And the chiropractic contention is that chiropractic conclusions are derived from biological science, but in disagreement in many areas with medical conclusions. This is what makes it free from the domination of medical allopathy.

In line with this trend to unite and solidify concepts along scientific lines, there are other current developments that are influencing the future of scientific chiropractic conclusions. Recently, for example, Roy W Hildebrandt, DC, editor of the JOURNAL of MANIPULATIVE and PHYSIOLOGICAL THERAPEUTICS, called attention to his analyzing that neither chiropractic nor medicine refer to themselves as a "science," but rather more accurately as a "discipline."

What might less technically be concluded from this observation would be an impression that studies can be entered into, "scientifically," but though there is a "science" of doing this and a "science" of doing that, it still does not add up to an actual, independent science.

There is no intended challenging of Dr Hildebrandt, for he does make an excellent point, here, in that medicine and chiropractic (both), as disciplines, would be more accurately classified as distinct "training" that would be intended as a means to incorporate such training into a branch of scientific knowledge, or scientific teaching.

Arguing against the contention that we should refrain from literally describing ourselves as a science, it might be stated that since the medical profession has no hesitancy in referring to itself as the practice of medical science, using this as a model of semantic reference, the chiropractic profession should feel just as secure in referring to itself, also, in this sense, as chiropractic science.

The final decision would still be debatable and based, probably, on whether the chiropractic profession exists as a science or, like medicine, is scientific because it employs scientific investigation, conclusions and procedures.

In commenting on the part played by chiropractic in the area of science as relating to practicing chiropractors, Frank P De Giacomo, DC, author of "Man's Greatest Gift to Man...CHIROPRACTIC," says "...it is not sufficient that a practice or technique or theory be scientific. It must be something more

3

than scientific." And he adds, "it is proven in the textbooks of neurology that man is a thoroughly integrated unit, that the nervous system is the integrating mechanism, and that it must be intact in order to function normally. This is a basic principle in chiropractic."

In positioning chiropractic relation to science, Dr De Giacomo further elaborates when he says, "It is just as scientific to consider structural cause of disease as to consider chemical cause, and most certainly cause is the thing in which the chiropractor is interested."

Dr De Giacomo, in his text, refers to the scientific laboratory in connection with "the leading role" played by the nervous system in the phenomena of health and disease and concludes, "...laboratory findings have confirmed the clinical observations of chiropractors, and it may be correctly stated that chiropractic is as much the outgrowth of the experimental method as any other science."

For a further full support being added to an illumination of the part being played by science in chiropractic in connection with its practice, you are referred to Chapter 12 of Dr De Giacomo's text, "Is Chiropractic a Science?"

In 1982, T L Shrader, DC called attention of the profession to a very profound 48-page booklet by C O Watkins, DC (The Basic Principles of Chiropractic Government). He described the book as "spelling out the formula as accurately and objectively as anything I have ever read. He considers the legal ramifications of a chiropractic, defined as a science, and granted the logical freedom to advance consistent with its principles and within the limits imposed by law.

"It is of inestimable value to grasp how the past and future discovery of physiological principles and ways to use them might fit into, and with, a dynamic, scientifically defined chiropractic profession.

"C O 'Pure Science' Watkins was an in-depth thinker, dedicated to the profession."

Dr Watkins has stated: "There are no absolute facts in science. A conclusion may be arrived at but only temporary. If a subsequent fact seems to dispute the conclusion, it is readily abandoned for what seems to be a more exact one. Science subscribes to no doctrine and sees no harm in reversing its position if new knowledge warrants it."

In commenting on the division of science employed in chiropractic education, Dr Watkins comments:

Chiropractic as Applied Science

The basic sciences of chiropractic (biology, anatomy, physiology, chemistry, hygiene, etc.) are not, strictly speaking, a part of the science of chiropractic. They are basic sciences. Chiropractic is an applied science. We should never forget that chiropractic is an applied science and of much more importance to us than the basic sciences. The science of chiropractic is our responsibility and ours alone."

Dr Watkins volunteers this caution in regard to chiropractic as a science, stating, "Chiropractic can be established and defended as a separate science only so far as we organize our own clinical research to find our own specific facts and general laws as they apply to chiropractic methods."

Editorially, Dr Watkins commented that chiropractic is regarded as a natural science -not as a super-natural science- by the average chiropractic physician, consequently, he has no need for either dogma or cult.

Dr Watkins recommended as one of the means to accomplish scientific organization, the program of organizing a nomenclature committee to standardize chiropractic, scientific terminology with a directive on chiropractic nomenclature then to be published.

Within the chiropractic realm, Dr T L Shrader has been one who has strongly supported these recommendations.

5

Authoritative observations

A little over ten years ago, a group of chiropractic educators headed by Helmut Bittner, DC got together to formulate a commentary on the chiropractic of that day. Members were: Doctors A Earl Homewood, William D Harper, Joseph J Janse, and C W Weiant. Commenting on "Chiropractic as Science," they had this to say:

"Chiropractic is a body of classified knowledge. The essentials of the basic sciences form the nucleus of chiropractic education. From the basic sciences come the data which support the theory of chiropractic and shape the practice. Such knowledge is supplemented by additional knowledge garnered from chiropractic centres in various parts of the world.

"Chiropractic represents the typical attitude characteristic of science. There is within chiropractic an insatiable curiosity concerning the phenomena with which its practitioners deal. There is a willingness to modify any theory when more tenable explanations are advanced and to abandon error when error is shown to exist. There is a definite disposition also to demonstrate the efficacy of chiropractic by subjecting it to comparative evaluation, using other therapies as controls. The methods of obtaining data in chiropractic are the methods of science. These include: Observation and description, experimentation, and statistics."

And the group ended their commentary with this observation:

"Chiropractic is stringently bound by the rules of logic. It reasons by induction and deduction, applies the methods of establishing causal relations and follows accepted procedures in formulating hypotheses and theories."

T F Ratledge, DC, a highly-respected chiropractic educator, described chiropractic as being a branch of biological science and entering into scientific conclusions since our observations and conclusions were based on the conclusions of biological science.

For purposes of this text, it would be safe in referring to the chiropractic profession as being engaged in the practice of scientific chiropractic. And it will be a purpose of this text to help establish such conclusion.

Birth of a Science

T F Ratledge, who was a contemporary of D D Palmer, invited Dr Palmer to be associated with his school that was later known as Ratledge Chiropractic College. Dr Ratledge had known and visited with the Palmer family for several years, but it was at this time that the two had an opportunity to engage in many long discussions in connection with the birth and development of chiropractic as a science. Here, then, in the words of Dr Ratledge, is an account of how chiropractic came into existence as a science through the intellectual and persistent efforts of D D Palmer.

"In the year 1895, a man with an inquiring mind and tremendous courage, a student of nature and natural law, human life and its manifestations of health, sickness and death, his mind untrammeled by the chaos of superstitious beliefs that were generally accepted as facts -many of which are still so-accepted- did much personal and private research in the area of mysterious forces. There were magnetism, hypnotism, combustion, electricity, mind power and force, innate potential forces in the human body. And some of these forces must, he believed, initiate and influence the mechanical, chemical and thermal manifestations of the body under all conditions. He actually attempted -and for a brief period thought he was- practicing magnetism.

"It was during this period that he observed what appeared to be frequent irregularities in the vertebral columns of different patients. However, he was particularly impressed with the striking fact that he could find no demonstrable evidence of any alleged diseases.

"This was a thought which he admitted to me was frightening, at first. But by further research, he was definitely and fully convinced that the idea was supported by the rules of

7

logic and all known and established biological facts in weighing the discovery of this vertebral irregularity in patients related to ill health.

"It became his conviction that he would stand on his own opinion, irrespective of what society might think of him or what calumny might be heaped upon him by the medically educated and prejudiced scientists whose utterances were made public opinion.

"Organized medicine soon became aware of chiropractic science and the profession. However, the principle of the Golden Rule and individual freedom, as established under the Constitution of the United States has defeated medical politicians, thus guaranteeing the freedom of choice in selecting the health service in which they believe.

"Other countries have now followed the American pattern and made the health service of chiropractic science available to their peoples, far and wide, throughout the world.

"When Dr D D Palmer realized the vicious nature of medical attacks against chiropractic approval by state legislatures, he knew that a life and death political struggle between the science of chiropractic and superstitions was imminent. Wishing to avoid a negative discussion of medical history and existing status, he decided to do research into the general scientific --and questionable-- accomplishments of medical practice. He turned, first, to medical literature. He then turned to libraries, vigorously searching for recorded alleged facts of medical successes in the common diagnosed diseases.

' In discussing the general subjects of human health and sickness with his fellow scientist researchers, Dr Palmer observed that he had been unable to find even one instance of an approved and recorded cure for any disease whatsoever. Each of his associated researchers reported the same results.

"There have never been but two concepts of human sickness. The first was what has developed into today's practice of medicine. The second concept resulted from Dr D D Palmer's repeated scientific demonstrations of the overall importance of the human nerve system as the sole instigator, regulator, coordinator and perpetuator of all cellular and organic functional activity that may occur in the human body.

"The natural type of energy or force arising in and projected by and from stimulated nerve cells eluded many research scientists until Dr Palmer ascertained that it was of an electric type and required special channels which are extensions of similar substance as that of which the cell body is composed.

"In considering the nerve system his research determined that nerve energy is a stimulus. It provides a perfect provision for exciting and coordinating the activities of all functional cells in the human body, and as long as the cells are adequately nourished (and there is no obstruction to appropriate transmission), functioning will be sufficient to mai ntain a normal, or tolerable environment and the body will experience life and good health."

Ratledge concepts

T F Ratledge was a chiropractic educator for nearly fifty years. In protesting against those aspects of medicine toward which he was negatively impressed, Dr Ratledge naturally described the area of chemistry as an exact science, --which is irrefutable. The basic lack of science in general medicine, however, he described as being due to the assumption of knowing the chemistry of the human body while it is in the process of perpetual change, even fluctuating with every inspiration and every expiration that constantly affects it.

Dr T F Ratledge, like Dr BJ Palmer and so may others at the time, carried a rabid anti-medicine attitude to the point of being so intent upon exposing that which was objectionable about the practice of medicine that they lashed out at all MDs. But Dr Ratledge was dedicated to an enlightening of the world

9

to an appreciation of the facts of chiropractic science. And on the continuing pages of this text will be found not only the wisdom of D D Palmer/Willard Carver-inspired Ratledge conclusions but the updated additional advancements from ongoing scientific investigation and demonstration.

Dr T F Ratledge insisted that the scientific practice of chiropractic be divorced from any consideration of it as limited to being just a specialty. And in further evaluating chiropractic he wanted to assure the world as to limitations that exist when engaged only in symptomatic care. He emphasized that scientific chiropractic teaches that symptoms of ill health are actually just exactly what the human body, itself, would and does, manifest under the various environmental influences to which the tissues may be subjected.

Dr Ratledge was satisfied that every symptom is readily understood with a sufficient knowledge of the anatomical structure and functioning of the tissues of the body.

With such a degree of uniqueness about scientific chiropractic, it has been contended that chiropractic science should have a vocabulary of its own. The facts are that chiropractic science has, definitely, introduced a vocabulary that has brought a vocabulary of its own. The facts are that chiropractic science has, definitely, introduced a vocabulary that has brought about changes in accepted understanding by the scientific community as a consequence of chiropractic development of more descriptive language.

Chiropractic principles make themselves known as a revision to medical theorizing as chiropractic terminology begins to educate and to enlighten as to the very nature of the chiropractic concept. This is why an understanding of chiropractic terminology is so very important in any consideration of chiropractic science.

Chapter II

PRINCIPLES

History

The history of dealing with the subject of chiropractic principles has been one that has been open to interpretation and reinterpretation throughout the years.

In most instances, there has been a tendency to be overly philosophical, in the past, when considering the form in which chiropractic principles have been presented.

There has been a reason for that - as will be seen as the message of this chapter unfolds.

One of the first recognized texts designed to inform the student in connection with formulated chiropractic principles was published in 1927 and authored by R W Stephenson, DC, Palmer faculty member. His CHIROPRACTIC TEXTBOOK listed thirty-three principles of chiropractic and started off in a philosophical sense, dealing with existence of and activities of a universal intelligence as a major premise.

Original Principles

In the matter of original principles, A Earl Homewood, DC, well known as an educator in both Canada and the United States, in his text, THE NEURODYNAMICS OF THE VERTEBRAL SUBLUXATION, comments:

...it is necessary to constantly quote from the works of D D Palmer to establish the exact principles and separate them from the peculiar ideas and theories from the fertile brains of others. Many of these latter theories do not stand with the light of present day knowledge, yet the teaching of D D Palmer will be found consistent with the facts of our present

11

stage of intellectual insight and are likely to be found capable of withstanding investigation in the light of new knowledge yet to be discovered -for these are basic truths and principles..

With the knowledge and assurance that the basic principles of chiropractic are sound and correct, there need be no qualms regarding critical investigation of the theory. Nor can any theory, based upon the known facts of today, be expected to stand unchanged for posterity...

It may be assumed that any theory, based upon facts, could be as useful for one school of chiropractic thought as another. The nervous system acts upon one set of laws and the knowledge of those laws will explain the reason for the efficaciousness of the varied methods of application of the basic principles of chiropractic. Each chiropractor may create, or modify, his methods and each technique be effective, providing it is the application of a true principle...

...clinical results have proven the truth of the chiropractic principle to the extent that most critics and biased persons are forced to admit the benefits to be derived from the techniques used by chiropractors. [End of quote]

D D Palmer

D D Palmer referred to the "principles which compose the science" of chiropractic. He described science as the "accepted, accumulated knowledge, systematized and formulated with reference to the existence of general facts –the operation of general laws concerning one subject." And in describing chiropractic as a science, he called attention to its existence as a consequence of existing principles when he said, "Chiropractic is the name of a classified, indexed, knowledge of successive sense impressions of biology --the science of life-- which science I created out of principles which have existed as long as the vertebrata."

D D Palmer described chiropractic as being explained "by the understanding of the principles."

12

In D D Palmer's day, he not only described scientific chiropractors as being "versed in the principles of chiropractic," he added that "They live according to its rules."

Under the heading of these principles, he referred to the relieving of pressure on nerves in order to allow a "transmitting and receiving of impulses to and from the various parts of the body in a normal manner."

D D Palmer said the principles that compose chiropractic "are substantive in their independence and incentive to human and spiritual progress."

From the above, you can see that the originator of chiropractic as a science was pretty well caught up in establishing the importance of principles, –where they relate to chiropractic science in the initial stages of his organizing it.

D D Palmer, in these initial stages, having previously been involved with the health states of people in which he was conscious of their variations in debility or strength, naturally, described himself as being very interested in the part played by what he called, at the time, "tone," in relation to the health of the individual.

At the time, he even went so far as to describe this "tone" as the "basic principle, the one from which all other principles, which compose the science, have sprung."

So even though we rarely hear reference to this original declaration of D D's that he considered tone as of such importance that he thought of it as a basic principle, today's chiropractic has reconstructed and revised this concept, during its period of evolving as a science, and in adding to this original concept has brought it up to the more appropriate understanding that fits into today's expanded knowledge.

In referring to this, it must not be in the sense of playing down that original premise of Dr D D Palmer. There was a continuity at the time that must be taken into consideration so that there will be no act of taking this concept out of context with what Dr Palmer had been involved with at the time and was further developing. There should not be a failure to appreciate the need for such conclusion at this time when the original concept was shaping up.

A few short years after the death of D D Palmer in 1913, with the influence of BJ Palmer and others there was a dropping of the attention that had been directed toward the term, tone. The BJ Palmer concentration upon the Innate concept tended to direct more attention to this than to the original tone-oriented manner of reference.

Tone and tonicity of tissues

Later on, in the '30s, particularly, there was a replacement for this tone concept and chiropractic education in some instances directed attention to what was referred to as the tonicity of tissues, but in a lesser degree than expressed by D D, originally. This was during a period when palpation was a more exacting art in chiropractic practice, and chiropractic students were impressed with the need to take into consideration the tonicity of the tissues being examined. This was noted as an essential element of observation and helped the practicing doctor to determine to what degree functioning was contributing to healthy tissues or unhealthy tissues.

William D Harper, DC, Dean Administrator of Texas Chiropractic College at the time he authored a text subtitled as a "Correlation of Dr Daniel David Palmer's PRINCIPLES of CHIROPRACTIC," addressed this subject of tone under the sub-head, Tone or Irritability:

"If we go back to D D Palmer (1,p.352) we find the following as the basis of this science: 'I founded the science of chiropractic upon the basic principle of tone. By reasoning upon the immutable laws of biology, which are based upon tone, the living principle of animal and vegetable life.' He further adds: 'The quality of irritability gives tone.' This was his first principle. Therefore, the foundation of the principles of chiroprac-

14

tic lies in the property of irritability of protoplasm."

Dr Harper enlarged upon this concept when he quoted Starling in his Physiology: "The whole study (of physiology) must be based on the existence of consciousness in all living things as well as in ourselves. This property of consciousness or awareness of environmental change has its basis in the property of irritability of protoplasm."

Dr Harper further enlarges on the subject by remarking, "This introduces the idea of cellular as well as organism consciousness." And, of course, it is with this modernized version that we begin to get into what chiropractic science has been developing in accordance with the revelations of biological science.

This will be developed further in later chapters.

Having found it necessary, for purposes of recording the historical implications related to D D Palmer's originating chiropractic as a science and placing emphasis, at the time, upon what he then considered as essential principles, there is now a need to make reference to the subject by quoting a page right out of D D Palmer's original text on Chiropractic, printed in 1910, relating the actual wording used by Dr Palmer:

TONE

The basic principle of the science and philosophy (not the art) of Chiropractic is tone, a word of four letters, yet it comprises a whole thot, a complete sentence; grammatically it is entire, inasmuch as it expresses a complete thot...

A basic principle is the foundation, the source, the origin, that from which other principles may proceed, or are derived.

The science and philosophy of Chiropractic is built on tone. The source of every Chiropractic principle, whether physiological or pathological, is founded upon tone. That one word means much to a Chiropractor who desires to comprehend the basis of Chiropractic in its scientific or philosophical phase.

Tone is that state or condition of a body, or any of its organs or parts in which the organic or animal functions are performed with due vigor.

The tone or tension of muscles and organs or firmness of nerves, muscles or organs, the renitent, elastic force acting against an impulse. Any deviation from normal tone, that of being too tense or too slack, causes a condition of renitence, too much elastic force, too great resistance, a condition expressed in function as disease.

Tonicity, or tone, is a quality belonging to solids; it is normal when the tension or partial contraction of nerves and muscles is at rest.

All life, vegetable or animal, depends upon tone, for its normal or abnormal existence...

Tone is the basic principle upon which I founded the science and developed the philosophy of Chiropractic. [End of quote]

Interestingly, with that enthusiastic statement made by D D, the subject then seems to do a fade-out and dwindle down to only two more references within the pages of the rest of the entire 1007-page D D Palmer Chiropractor's Adjuster.

On page 841, D D asks, "What is tone?" His answer: "Normal tension."

The final reference to tone is made on page 971:

"Tone is elasticity and renitency of tissue which responds to compression.

"The renitency of tissue is the inherent quality of life, the ability to resist pressure. In biology, it is the condition resulting from elastic force acting against an impulse. The elastic force of nerves furnishes the momentum of impulses. This innate quality of springing back, recovering its normal size, shape and position is known as tone. Hence, we have nerve tone, muscle tone, arterial tone, etc. meaning the ability of those tissues to assume, return to their normal position, size and shape after being acted upon by pressure.

"It is a self-evident fact that any change in tissue other than that of normal tension, produces disease, tone being the product of elasticity and renitency.

"The distinctive character of tone is due to tension...

"...For all practical purposes, (tension) is estimated by palpation with the fingers...'

So the subject of tone as a principle, as dealt with by D D Palmer, in chiropractic's early day period, being given emphasis by D D in relation to chiropractic principles, is referred to, here, not to suggest returning to that early-day period for literal incorporation into today's concepts, –but to illustrate how original concepts have served their purpose, been added to and become advanced into today's concepts without detracting from their originally conceptualized area of importance.

Changes

The fundamental thought in these original concepts is still there, but somewhere along the line it became necessary to modernize such reference and bring it up to date, making such changes as would be necessary for positioning this original concept into more harmonious agreement with today's knowledge. And this is what the chiropractic profession and its representatives have done and are doing as an ongoing evidence of their capability to recognize the value of keeping up to date.

An idea, when it is first introduced, can have tremendous impact. It is new. There is knowledge-expansion attention being directed toward it. And people are conscious of thought-revisions being set in motion because of it. But then comes a slackening off of interest. As that idea takes hold and begins to influence more associated thought, with even newer ideas added, the original idea then becomes more commonplace and loses that original impact. It is now older. It has been accepted over a period of time. It has lost some of its quality of attractability. People are now dealing with what has developed as an outcome of that original idea.

Today

If D D Palmer were alive today, he would have now brought his early thoughts more up to date because it has been shown he was a man who continued to investigate further as a true scientific-minded researcher. And where he made reference to "tone," in the beginning, he would now be more inclined to have added newer knowledge and, no doubt, be inclined to state that what he now had in mind in regard to "tone" represented the very fundamental existence of life within the body but also incorporated an understanding of homeostasis and the fact that life expresses itself through matter in a recognizable manner that allows us to take certain chiropractic steps, based upon biological principles that cooperate with natural law to help restore anatomical functioning, satisfactorily. And he would probably continue to refer to the inherent properties of living organisms that distinguish them in such manner that they must be considered in all aspects of satisfactory health recovery.

There has been a period of over eighty years, now, during which there has been an opportunity to conjecture over what the intent of D D Palmer would have been in continuing his introductory phase of chiropractic understanding, allowing a continuity of his intended revelations and refinement of his original concepts.

In considering the part played in the adjustive processes related to improving transmission of nerve impulses, here, again, he has shown that though, necessarily, starting with experimental adjusting procedures, he would now, naturally, be supporting the newer knowledge and developments that have allowed expansion of his original ideas. But he would have no reason to tamper with his original recognition of the biological principle that incorporated the fact that there can be interference with nerve transmission to the point of interfering with the state of health and that good health would, automatically, return when the corrections were made to allow good health restoration.

So the point here is that there were, definitely, biological principles that were considered when chiropractic was born as a science, through D D Palmer's organizing it as such. And those biological principles maintain, today, so that chiropractic can continue on as a specific discipline of recognized science.

Chiropractic is evolving. And recognizing and joining in with the ongoing developments of science will help it to further evolve.

Osteopathic principles

To illustrate a point, further, it might be mentioned that in the case of osteopathy, while its originator, Dr Andrew T Still, was alive, there was an understanding, such as the understanding that has been carried on in the chiropractic profession by respecting the D D Palmer concepts, to the effect that what Dr Still taught was supported by principles upon which he elaborated. But in the late 1950s, it was reported in connection with the annual osteopathic convention that there was an evident playing down of osteopathic principles. It was like a turning point. Osteopathy was entering a phase of change. It was now more medical-oriented.

Editorially, there is a constant warning to the chiropractic profession not to allow this same departure from principles to happen to chiropractic as was instrumental in emasculating the drugless program of early-day osteopathy.

Science or philosophy

In searching for just a single, basic, scientific principle that

19

would attach itself to what it is the chiropractic physician is governed by in his/her conclusions, it would have to be the more commonly-accepted one that has been expressed in a varied number of ways, yet retains the concept that there can be an interference with the delivery of neurological messages, discoverable and correctible through chiropractic procedures, affecting the health of the individual. This, of course, would be in the sense of establishing a scientific principle based upon recognition of biological science.

It is when we get into the philosophical realm that there enters an area of conjecture over conclusions. The philosophical deals to a large extent with a consideration of the intricacies of how a "life force" becomes a concern for chiropractic consideration and arouses conjecture as to why activities manifest themselves in the manner in which they appear to do so.

The philosophical concept is still there as an influence in connection with further developing the chiropractic concept, but what the profession has been slow to recognize is that whereas the concept originally looked to philosophy to explain it, -because there was a need at the time to incorporate such a wholehearted effort in order to accomplish certain purposes-, there now has arrived an opportunity to base the chiropractic concept more securely on scientific fundamentals without detracting from those instances where the concept can be further supported by philosophical conjecturing.

A concern for principles

Taking a cue from others outside the chiropractic profession, one hears the words of the respected author, Pearl S Buck:

"It is no simple matter to pause in the midst of one's maturity, when life is full of function, to examine what are the principles which control that functioning." This thought particularly applies to chiropractic's current status of maturity in regard to concern for principles.

20

Yesterday and today

The profession seems too caught up 'in the midst of one's maturity' in technical and other aspects of functioning to devote very much attention to the area of studious concern for standardized acceptance of what would be concluded to be basic chiropractic principles. But in D D Palmer's time it was different. There was time for considering and mulling over philosophical and scientific principles. And people, at that time, in their slower-paced living, were finding the subject an area of major importance for keen concern.

A love for principles

A comment on principles attributed to the philosopher, Confuscious (556-479 BC), was the observation that 'He who merely knows right principles is not equal to him who loves them.' And this is most apropos, here, because it makes the comparison more understandable in considering the men and their times, such as D D Palmer and his contemporary, T F Ratledge, when they demonstrated such an intense 'love for' principles that their whole makeup and philosophy seemed dependent upon establishing the value of these concepts related to principles.

It may be that, today, we are not so much neglecting the area of principles as finding ourselves caught up in such endless distractions as to prevent our wholehearted participation in such as did those early pioneers of chiropractic fundamentals.

Influences

D D Palmer and T F Ratledge lived in a period when there was popular concern for 'divine and eternal principles' that influenced their thinking, at the time, and influenced their need to concentrate on making principles serve to explain and support their philosophical contentions. Under the heading of principles, they were respected for illuminating concepts that, though bearing upon interpretation of biologically sound physiological aspects were misclassified under the head-

21

ing of philosophy.

This fascination with concentration upon principles was undoubtedly influenced by the fact that in the period when D D
Palmer was putting together chiropractic basics, people were
more dependent upon the philosophical and were, more regularly than today, exposed to the prevalence of sermons that
directed attention to the dependence upon principles provided
by the Bible, itself, for instance. These were the "divine and
eternal" principles that were part of one's daily living.

It was all very much in order. But it was part of the beginning
of the century in time episode and not what we are, currently,
experiencing and being called upon to focus intense attention
toward in this period in which we are now nearing the end of
the century. It is no longer a time when doctors are being called upon to crusade to convince legislators, for example, that
this discovery of unique principles is a basis for separate licensing.

Necessity

Stating a basic principle in connection with chiropractic, in
its early days, is what allowed chiropractic to prove it was not
infringing upon the practice of medicine, or any other auxiliary medical practice, and was justified in declaring itself eligible for acceptance as a unique and necessary profession.

Security in principles

We shouldn't fear that new principles will be created to eliminate chiropractic as a science. The principles will not be created. They will be discovered. And with their discovery, if the
basic tenets of chiropractic are correct, they will endure and
prosper by the addition of any improvements to come through
research and discovery of added knowledge.

The revelation of a scientific truth (such as disclosure that
matter, for example, as we ordinarily think of it, is not solid
form but is an expression of varying vibratory rates), could be

22

included into our basic chiropractic principle without necessitating any change in, or addition of, a new principle that would alter our original concept.

As with all sciences, we have enlarged our concepts. We have expanded our knowledge.

Modification

The words of caution of Virgil Thomson should be considered, here. They lend a bit of wisdom in his remark: "The clearest statement of principle goes bad if it is repeated too often. It ceases to be a statement and becomes a slogan."

Historically, it can probably be shown that even D D Palmer, after his original concentration upon what he called "tone," developed enough additional information to influence his interweaving of this thought and enlarging it so that its original manner of presentation became modified. So the idea, itself, has not really been lost. It has just been incorporated into the developing concepts that have evolved into a different, and more acceptable, manner of presentation.

Sensitivity

Jacques Barzum at one time observed, "In any assembly, the simplest way to stop the transacting of business and split the ranks is to appeal to principle." And perhaps this is one of the reasons that in the necessity to establish a justifiable principle we have experienced such difficulty in asserting such in an all-out effort in the ranks of chiropractic present-day makeup.

Re-examination

In the matter of continued respect for what D D Palmer put together under the heading of principles, it was the author, Anne Morrow, wife of Charles Lindbergh, who commented to the effect that in considering changes of a fundamental nature it did not mean "abandoning our fundamental principles, but rather a reexamination to determine whether we are following the dead letter or the living spirit which they embody." And that is what the following has as a proposal in surveying the overall aspects that relate chiropractic to its principles.

It is not the purpose, here, to encourage an abandonment. It is a matter of exposing how our attitudes have come about and how we might reorganize to meet our present demands while retaining the best from what has been provided for us from the past.

Maintaining our principles that include the area of continued exploration to reassert our foundation that we maintain as being unique in that we subscribe to certain concepts should be an area that we should not neglect.

It should not remain for just the seemingly few philosophers to continually initiate interest along the lines of developing encouragement toward sustaining principles. It must be admitted that in today's concept such limited reference to tone as being all important would tend to give to current chiropractic an incomplete appearance of not taking into consideration all that has transpired in the chiropractic world since this original reference to tone.

Emotional respect

The natural respect for principles, as they relate to the birth of chiropractic as a science, is not dependent upon an emotional experience in which D D Palmer would be elevated to a position of infallibility in which it would be necessary to interpret his every word as though he had created a Chiropractic Bible for his faithful to, religiously, subscribe to as though his ideas of the time were meant to be taken as "Gospel" for all eternity. But it must be admitted that a certain amount of emotionalism –or even experiencing of respected qualities like love and admiration– could, understandably enter into this without blocking those necessary areas of depending upon the conclusions of the cold, hard facts of science. This has been the history of chiropractic, –a combining of the humanitarian considerations along with the scientific that enters into being concerned for the health of individuals.

Respect for what D D Palmer gave the world will not be diminished in accepting the fact that he was a great man and produced a revolutionary change in the approach to health matters as a historical change in a chain of continuing evaluation and reevaluation. But with such emotional regard for the man in connection with what he had done, depending upon a verbatim, continuing interpretation as an unchanging and unmodifiable concept, there would be no room left for the normal course of progress.

Chiropractic has evolved.

Principles have evolved.

If original principles can meet the test of time, they, too, will remain intact.

Examples

In chiropractic literature from the past, there can be found authors referring, sometimes, to the chiropractic principle and, sometimes, to chiropractic principles.

In the case of Jack E Ratledge, DC, son of Dr T F Ratledge, he referred to principles (in the plural) in this manner:

"The science of chiropractic is a definite and complete set of principles dealing with all biological phenomena. The science of chiropractic is distinct from all other 'biological concepts' and is characterized by the following:

"Chiropractic states that the environment and/or heredity, consisting of mechanical, chemical, thermal, photeric, electrical, psychical, sonic, etc. influences, all of which are the manifestations of the inviolate laws of physics and/or nature and/or universal intelligence, is the sole actuator of structural changes and function in protoplasm.

25

"Chiropractic states that the nerve system is the principle mechanism that attempts to coordinate one structure of the body with another and the body as an entity with the environment.

"Chiropractic states that any interference with the liberation and transmission of neural energy automatically and instantaneously decreases or abolishes the powers and properties of the body to respond to the various environmental factors.

"Chiropractic states that health is the inevitable manifestation of protoplasm that has adequately responded to environmental influences.

"The practice of chiropractic is the application of chiropractic principles."

Now, even though this satisfied Dr Jack Ratledge and others insofar as an interpretation of what his declarations incorporated as chiropractic principles, nevertheless, there are other considerations. There is the obvious awareness that graduates of other chiropractic colleges will tend to offer principles not incorporating the same wording, —though concluding along similar lines.

The point being established is that there can be variations in the matter of recognized chiropractic principles or premises. The fact is then evident that THE basic principle carries with it a basic understanding. This makes possible other principle-interpretations. They are interjected without detracting from what is described as the basic principle. And this basic principle is related to chiropractic interest in the nerve system, its functioning, and procedures in connection with conforming to an advanced understanding of this basic principle.

Conjecture as an example

The controversy over relating chiropractic to a principle, or to principles, can be further placed in position for weighing the pluses and minuses in considering a conjectural event:

26

Suppose someone decided to give the world a new science, today, based on a principle that declared that nerve receptors, when stimulated by appropriately voiced suggestion, will initiate a series of nerve impulses, from nerve to nerve, along nerve pathways, to influence function in a correspondingly appropriate response to aid in the restoration of health. And, of course, the practice of that science is naturally going to be known as "vocapractic" because the appropriate suggestion would issue from the voice. The voice procedure would be in accordance with the application of the basic principle.

It wouldn't be necessary to state all the other principles involved that could be incorporated into vocapractic. The main objective would be to establish that there was a science that would stand up to the test, based upon this primary principle, incorporating any other principles necessary to pursue this course. And if, after probable demonstrations of objections from both the medical and chiropractic professions, this science came through with public recognition and legislation for licensing, there would then be a newly established practice of a profession called vocapractic.

If there had been the added obstacle of being burdened with fighting to establish all the principles, then the originator would not have lasted even through the first round. And even if gaining the title, the chances of retaining it would be greater if there were fewer fights over the preliminaries of many supporting principles.

If other principles were included in the definition, there might come a time when the primary principle would be dropped and all that would be left would be those that served no value in justifying the existence as a separate and distinct science. Then vocapractic would have no unique purpose for existence. This, then, would seem to be an influential factor to prompt the supporting of a principle to serve as the foundation of practice of an accepted discipline or science.

Natural Law

T L Shrader, DC, a past President of the California Chiropractic Association, Secretary of the Chiropractic Forum and, currently, Secretary of the American Chiropractic Association Council on Technic, has expressed his thinking related to the recognition of chiropractic principles when he stated, "The chiropractic effort must be accurately based on a true principle of Natural Law to be worthy of our concern."

Dr Shrader, over the years, has encouraged a freedom of chiropractic thought designed not to limit conclusions just to what would be determined as chiropractic principle, solely from a single source, but has contended this should be open to more than one evaluation of what would constitute the basic principle. And he expressed it this way, "Those who are best grounded in principles closest to the truth have the best chance of success." And because he saw a need for bringing about better understanding in the area of questionable principles, he was an influential personality in organizing a Chiropractic Forum that served to explore and develop definitions and postulates related to the principle of chiropractic that might be more universally acceptable.

In an item for publication in 1982, Dr Shrader stated his impressions on the subject this way:

"Thank you for your invitation to discuss the topic of 'principles' with you and your readers of WORLD-WIDE REPORT. The subject needs consideration.

"We have all heard chiropractic spokespersons refer to the principle of chiropractic (singular). On occasion, reference is made to chiropractic principles (plural). When we are not sure even of the number of principles we claim, let alone uniformly agree upon their identity, then something is wrong.

"This has concerned me for many years. What effort I have periodically made to stimulate objective discussion either was rebuffed as unnecessary, or ignored, completely. Such reaction has led me to conclude, first, that many use the word, prin-

28

ciple, without knowing what it means; others have a vague idea but fail to realize how catastrophic the effect has been to let something upon which they claim to base their science to remain so imprecise.

"Lack of clear identity and lack of common purpose in our organizations is a direct result of our neglect in facing up to and resolving this issue.

"I have filing cabinets generously supplied with information on this topic. Some of the information was derived through field surveys conducted in the late forties and early fifties, --during our work with the Chiropractic Forum, in Los Angeles. One or several volumes could be written of the 'struggle on principles' which has intensely plagued this profession.

Reference

The impressive new text by Virgil V Strang, DC, Palmer Professor of Philosophy, "Principles of Chiropractic," does an excellent job in relating the basic chiropractic thinking in connection with the development of chiropractic principles and is a worthy candidate for the library of every chiropractic doctor and student. It is published by the Palmer College of Chiropractic.

Research

In connection with developments of the Chiropractic Forum, it was Allan D Le Vantine, DC who researched the area of chiropractic definition and, in doing so, found it necessary to clarify the relationship of the chiropractic principle concept.

What Dr Le Vantine concluded was that it was necessary to delve into the reason behind what is in the chiropractic principle in order to establish information as to the reason why chiropractic is what it is and why chiropractic does what it does.

Dr Le Vantine, in formulating his concept, concluded that

29

"reason" is really another expression for "principle." And under such conjecturing, it would follow that to find the principle upon which chiropractic is based, one asks "why?"

Dr Le Vantine made a very profound observation in this in-depth search for answers where chiropractic principle is concerned when he declared:

"The chiropractor has been educated by chiropractic in the principle of chiropractic even though he may not be able to reveal what that principle is." And Dr Le Vantine went on to further clarify by adding, "It is this principle that differentiates chiropractic and makes it unique among the several contestants in the health field." And, finally, Dr Le Vantine volunteers the observation that "Where other health sciences apply methods, chiropractic applies its principle. It is the stressing of the principle that makes chiropractic what it is."

Dr Le Vantine lists seventeen chiropractic premises that formulate what it is that chiropractic concepts contend and presume. And then he further clarifies by asserting that "these are the premises of chiropractic as expressed by the profession, --but they are not principles. They cannot be fitted into a definition. They express the thought and consideration that the chiropractor uses in his professional art, while considering its many facets, but the motivation for each of these premises is what we are really looking for.

"This motivation is the true reason or principle of chiropractic, as seen expressed in each of the seventeen premises."

Analyzing, this principle is more or less as follows:

"To establish proper conditions in both body and environment so that the body/environment relationship will be such that it will allow the inherent and natural forces of the body to bring about a satisfactory state of health."

Dr Le Vantine concludes:

30

"What we have solved is the reason or the true principle that stands as the motivating force to all of chiropractic. The principle tells why chiropractic does what it does but not how it does it."

Dr Le Vantine uses a positive attitude toward what he put together when he further concluded:

"The principle will serve as a 'yard stick' to stabilize the realm of chiropractic. It will show exactly which health procedures are chiropractic and which procedures are not, in the same manner that Lincoln's principle shows which procedures are representative of a democracy and which are not. Thus, the principle of chiropractic is found to be the ideological basis of an infallible definition of chiropractic."

Dr Le Vantine says accepting a premise as the principle is in error and adds, "Actually, there are many premises, but there is only one principle. Two factions, each accepting a different premise as the principle could never agree."

Questions

Is there an ultimate chiropractic authority, or authorities, on chiropractic principle, or principles? Or, do the principles represent something that has been passed along with never an out-and-out assertion and affirmation?

Was there ever a clear-cut statement of principles that could be formulated for all time, unvaried in its presentation, so that the chiropractic student, today, could rely upon this guideline?

Dependence

Most assuredly, chiropractic principles are taught in all chiropractic colleges. The important point is that they must continue to be taught, no matter what variations in wording. And such principles, to be scientifically acceptable, would have to exist within the understanding of biological science, itself, and have developed from such understanding.

It has been stated that it is through the application of chiropractic principles that the practicing doctor is in position to meet the varying demands of circumstances to which the doctor responds.

These chiropractic principles must be in the sense of affording direction in procedures that can be applied, consistently, to all conditions one meets.

It should be an understood essential consideration for any doctor to understand that it is necessary to deal with facts.

It is necessary to deal with matter and the laws that govern the activity of such matter. These are the laws that control all manifestations of living and non-living matter. And the need is to deal with the error of considering only the symptoms of disease, instead of relating directly to the function involved.

If that which is manifesting itself is explainable, then it should be self-evident that there will be exposed a true cause and a corresponding result, or effect.

The human body is really a simple thing when we really come down to its accurate consideration, though appearing complex.

Life cannot manifest itself except when the right combination of matter is provided in the environment. This combination takes the form of mechanical, chemical or thermal influences.

In a sense, the work of the medical physician is a form of first aid.

When the doctor has done for those in emergency situations what can be done for them, then recovery, itself, becomes dependent upon the power produced by and within the individual's body. In this sense, there is a dealing with the principle involved in such recovery.

By chiropracticly adjusting, the doctor is taking pressure off nerves. And it is because of the principle involved, here, that one concludes the necessity for vertebral adjustment.

Whatever the chiropractic doctor does to apply the principles having a bearing upon the concepts associated with chiropractic procedures to the widest extent, is proper.

Without referring to them, specifically, as "principles," throughout this text will be found the description of what are the guiding chiropractic concepts that, together, serve to make up the principles attached to chiropractic reasoning in coming to its overall conclusions.

Chapter III

RESEARCH

Introduction

In the European Journal of Chiropractic, June, 1984, volume 32, number 2, published by Blackwell Scientific Publications, there is this commentary on Research in Chiropractic by Robert T Anderson, PhD, DC, Professor of Anthropology, Mills College, Research Committee Chairman, California Chiropractic Association:

"The Foundation for Chiropractic Education and Research, an agency of the American Chiropractic Association, sponsored the Conservative Health Science Research Conference in Chicago... Twenty-six papers were read before the scientific audience... (There was a) new high in the level of research activity now taking place on problems relating to chiropractic... We all came away with a sense of the high scientific integrity of research programmes taking place all over the United States and Canada... Malcolm Pope, PhD, showed slides to show work being carried out in his university... James Miller, PhD, of the University of Illinois, reported on work performed in his laboratory relating to biomechanics of facets and spinal nerves. Two chiropractor researchers from the state laboratory, Dr John J Triano and Dr Sean Moroney, provided additional reports in the sessions... The University of Colorado was represented by Marvin Luttges, PhD, the University of Toronto and Canadian Memorial Chiropractic College by John Duckworth, MD, and McMasters University by Adrian Upton, MD... Oakland, California was the site of a second research conference held just 1 month later. Under the Chairmanship of Professor Chung-ha Suh of the University of Colorado, the occasion was the 14th Annual Biomechanics Conference of the Spine. The meeting was cosponsored by the Biomechanics Laboratory of the University of Colorado along with the International Chiropractors Association and Life Chiropractic College West."

The field of research within the chiropractic profession, while under way since its inception, includes a current area of concentrated attention throughout the academic field as well as in areas such as private practice, and this chapter will be dealing with such phases. But first, there will be the introduction of some of the important related basics.

Current overall considerations

As a preliminary to this chapter on research, it might be wise to, first, refer to a commentary of R Lee Kirby, MD, Faculty of Medicine, Dalhousie University, Halifax, Nova Scotia, Canada B3H 4K4, when he presents a critique of "The Scientific Method in the ARCHIVES of PHYSICAL MEDICINE REHABILITATION for February, 1984 and concerns himself with the methodology of scientific research reporting, today.

The article relates to inductive and deductive approaches and observes that the "Inductive inference from empirical observations has been a mainstay of the scientific method..." and then adds the thought that theorists have expressed doubts about the exclusive use of the inductive approach, arguing an impossibility of true verification. The reference is to knowledge as mere accumulated perceptions.

Deduction, referring to formal logic, is drawing conclusions from ones premises. But unconscious assumptions can color these premises, says the author.

Deductive logical reasoning, however, allows a discovery of what our theories imply.

There is a moving onward from one hypothesis acting as a guide.

The author suggests that going for the weakest point, rather than, customarily, the strongest point, might be a more successful approach. And he adds that it has been observed that "if one examines the actual methods employed by great scientists, their research looks more like the opportunistic tactics of guerilla warfare than the organized strategies of major combats."

It has been suggested that a change be instituted that would "no longer rule out essential gambits of actual science."

The conclusion is that there should be concentration more on the area of "research program" than on individual theories.

The author makes a plea for a research program that "would consist of both hard-core fundamental, highly corroborated assumptions and a series of theories where each subsequent theory results from adding auxiliary clauses to the previous one."

By some, the term, "scientific paradigm" is used and suggested that "normal science" will prevail when the majority of scientists accept the same paradigm.

The paradigm is referred to as "highly immune to falsification."

The scientific method is referred to as "a concept in evolution."

The conclusion is that there is a need to test objective conclusions as severely as possible.

So it can be seen that the scientific method of research, itself, is under pressure for possible acceptance of new concepts in the scientific approach.

Neurological knowledge

In the case of chiropractic science, research should include among other factors the ascertainment of what nerve energy is, its origin and influence upon cells to which it may be conducted, and the reasons for failure of its transmission.

Obstruction affecting function

Obstruction. resulting from pressure upon nerves, regardless of diameter of nerve fibers or how many fibers may be in a nerve or nerve tissue involved and diminished energy production, are the most important causes of functional failure and the resulting organic -or tissue– manifestations. Such conclusions have come from research. Perhaps this has not been what we would classify as formal research, but, nevertheless, it has been the conclusions of research.

Need for terminology

In the pursuit of research, it would seem imperative that scientific chiropractic formulate and employ a distinctive terminology that would be designed to accurately express chiropractic thought as distinguished from medical terminology that can only foster medical conclusions.

Forms of research

Chiropractic physicians, in their personal practice offices are engaged, every day, in a form of research. And when their findings are collectively submitted, it will show support for the chiropractic premise.

Small scale research

An example of current efforts to increase the tempo of growing interest in clinical research can be illustrated by referring to what is developing in Stockton, California.

A Stockton Foundation for Chiropractic Research has been instituted at the office of Dr Don D Smallie, 2027 Grand Canal Boulevard. It is a non-profit group action.

Instrumental in organizing along scientific lines is the direction of Joseph C Keating, Jr, PhD, of the Department of Psychology at University of Pacific and associated with the Research Department of Palmer College of Chiropractic/WEST, in Sunnyvale, California.

The current project of the Foundation involves "Chiropractic

Care for Patients with Chronic Headache: An Experimental Test of Efficacy."

The intent is to provide chiropractic care, without cost to patients who have been suffering from chronic headache for at least one year, receiving no relief or only partial relief from medication.

The program includes orientation-briefing and monitoring, baseline, chiropractic care, early follow up, and one year follow-up.

Commenting on the small-scale, controlled chiropractic project, Dr Keating observes: "Without delving into the historical, political professional, and financial reasons for the paucity of chiropractic outcome research, suffice it to say that current circumstances allow for collaborative studies among chiropractors and a variety of other health-care professionals. The social environment of health-care sciences at present encourages interdisciplinary efforts to understand and influence CNS control of human physiology."

Increasing optimism

It was the experience of Dr Ratledge that there has been a tendency to greatly underestimate the power of the human body to recover from injury and degeneration of cells. However, he stated that in chiropractic education there is no evidence of underestimating such power as is the case in the study of medicine.

He further insisted there has been unwarranted pessimism concerning some of the more serious conditions manifested by the body, and he was very aware that many chiropractors refuse to serve individuals and refer them to other professions instead of bringing to bear every known bit of chiropractic knowledge, first, before capitulating to a referal before all factors had been considered.

Research has shown that chiropractic principles, applied in practice, are imperative in every instance for complete recovery from illness of such degree that the vital cellular degeneration is of such degree that recuperation is slower than required for acute or immediately recent functional impairment, or for recovery in the shortest possible time from acute conditions.

Cells, like batteries, may degenerate to such degree that they cannot be restored to normal metabolic and functional state, but Dr Ratledge voiced a concern that the chiropractic doctor too hastily concludes that degenerative degrees manifest them·selves as irremedial more often than is the case.

Dr Ratledge was convinced that there is no condition of human tissues in which freeing nerves from obstructive pressures has not, at least, a holding effect, slowing degenerative processes in cells in general or in local areas. And, of course, he admitted that when functioning in a restricted area has been sufficiently impaired, and for a long enough period, certain cells may become so advanced in degenerative processes that recovery is impossible. Then, and then only, said Dr Ratledge, may surgery be advisable.

The health field is divided by two lines of thought. One of these lines of thought concludes that perfection in the human body in the matter of living, growing, self-maintenance, the power of recovery and from any adaptation to wide variations in the mechanical, chemical and thermal states of its environment is the source and nature of which all injury and all degress of injury arise.

Modern scientific research has discovered much, previously unknown, about different forms, or manifestations, of energy and their uses.

Nerve energy and coordination

The most immediately important energy is nerve energy which normally provides for the excitation of all functional, or working, cells of the body through which the chemistry, temperature and pressures within the human body are made, maintained and/or restored to normal. And further, coordinating all functioning within the body, heart, blood vessels, lungs,

39

glandular, muscular, brain, mental and sensory responses is accomplished by the fact of adequate production and transmission of this energy, -the exclusive product of nerve cells.

Nerve energy is a form of electro-magnetic, transmissible energy, generated in "nerve cells" which are widely and numerously distributed through the human body as disclosed by anatomical and functional observations. However, nerve cells are completely grouped in and are the chief constituent of-- gray matter of the brain, spinal cord and ganglia, the cells of the latter being similar to those found in the brain and spinal cord.

Nerve cells constitute one of the three classifications of functional cells and are the source of nerve energy which is the sole means providing for coordinate functioning of cells involved in mental processes, muscular and glandular action, upon the results of which the continuance of living itself and the state of individual health depends.

Discoveries

In the light of modern research discoveries, it is necessary that the structures and functioning of the human body be revised and reinterpreted.

Research by chiropractic science has shown that there is only one nerve system in a human body. And this nerve system is the only nerve means of coordinating the billions of functional cells of the human body in maintaining health.

Nerve energy is the exclusive product of stimulated nerve cells.

Modern research scientists now classify stimuli as primary or secondary. This means that the direct stimulatory influence of the innate qualities of environmental matter upon cells is primary, while the energy released from the sensory nerve cells stimulate the intermediate nerve cells and on to their dendrites of which their axones are distributed, proving beyond doubt that nerve impulses do stimulate, --but are always secondary and do not reside or occur in the environmental matter.

40

In chemical research, the most important result seems to be discovering just how much of a given chemical may be tolerated by the average person without apparent injury.

Cranial mechanisms

In the area of specific investigations that have recently been under way, representing chiropractic research, one of chiropractic's own, Robert T Anderson, DC, PhD, reported in the March, 1983 issue of WORLD-WIDE REPORT:

"Cranially oriented practitioners claim to identify minute movements in skull bones or in the entire cranial vault in both juvenile and adult patients. Until the last few years, no scientific research existed to verify these claims. This circumstance is changing.

"At the last annual Biomechanics Conference on the Spine, sponsored by the Biomechanics Laboratory of the University of Colorado, I reported on my own exploration into spheno-occipital relationships. My findings were consistent with cranial theory, although they should not be interpreted as having proved it.

"Working in the osteology laboratory of the University of California, Berkeley, I measured angular relationships at the articulation of the sphenoid with the occiput in 250 American Indian skulls. The sphenoid was found to be rotated in one-third of the specimens. The maximum range of angulation was 8 degrees. It should be noted that these are fairly substantial ranges of angulation.

"Far more impressive than my simple project is some of the work that has come out of the biomechanics laboratory of the College of Osteopathic Medicine of Michigan State University. Ernest Retzlaff, PhD, and his associates undertook histological studies of the parieto-parietal suture in mature but small squirrel monkeys. This investigation made it clear that in these adult primates this suture does not fuse.

"This provides a valuable clue to cranial mechanisms, since

41

anthropologists as well known as Ashley Montagu teach that in Homo sapiens this suture begins a slow process of fusion that begins around age 20 and is normally completed during the third decade.

"...Retzlaff and his fellow team members were able to measure bone movement under normal physiologic circumstances. It does occur.

"The single most impressive project carried out in this laboratory was undertaken by John E Upledger, DO. Dr Upledger attempted to document the subjective impressions of craniosacral mechanics reported by clinicians. To this end, he measured changes by recording bioelectric activity utilizing electromyography, electrocardiography and strain-gauge recordings or respiratory activity. The changes were measurable.

"The most recent contribution in this fascinating area was made by a specialist in orthopedic dentistry, Stephen P Broderson, DDS, a private practitioner in Berkeley, California. Last August, he published his study of movement in two patients as it resulted from treatment with the May splint, a mandibular repositioning pivotal appliance used in correcting misalignments of the tempero-mandibular joint (TMJ).As measured on pre- and post- x-rays, as well as on facebow mounted models. Dr Broderson demonstrated a substantial repositioning of the temporal and frontal bones relative to the maxilla.

"An enormous amount of research still needs to be carried out. That done so far, however, has been supportive of the basic claim that cranial bones can indeed move in post-adolescent years."

Ongoing developments

In 1971, Dr T L Shrader, warned the technic departments of all chiropractic colleges:"The pressure for chiropractic research cannot be ignored."And about this time,Congress provided NIH funds toward a ten-year research period. The continuing

42

study has been one of chiropractic at the University of Colorado under the direction of Chung H Suh, PhD, Chairman of Engineering Design.

Says Dr Suh, "My chiropractic related spinal biomechanical research began in 1969. We accomplished a great deal and published some of the findings. Our findings are documented and published every year. These publications contain several hundred pages, including photographs, research methodology and our results. The University of Colorado accepts this as chiropractic research...

"Today, scientists see that we have established a strong basic science position for chiropractic and chiropractors are interested in the scientific method. Times change, attitudes improve.

"We are successfully meeting the challenge from the scientific community...

"We have the potential to not only prove the effectiveness of chiropractic care but to accelerate and improve the chiropractic contribution to the health care delivery system. At the University, we have developed computer software that chiropractors can use in their own offices and clinics that is compatible with the enormous amount of information in the University's computer system. In that way chiropractors can offer their patients the most up to date computer aided x-ray analysis of the vertebral subluxation complex that is available. They can communicate to the University computer through the use of floppy disks. with each patient's particular vertebral subluxation complex that is available. They can communicate to the University computer through the use of floppy disks, with each patient's particular vertebral subluxation complex and receive exact instructions as to appropriate care.

"There is ongoing research being conducted on the neuropathophysiological component of the vertebral subluxation complex as well as the nervous system. We are working on what the vertebral subluxation is in the first place as well as its many causes. We are researching what chiropractic offers the health care delivery system –the vertebral subluxation complex and its effective care and prevention. To us, chiropractic research is vertebral subluxation research.

"The vertebral subluxation is very real. We have documented it again and again. With this scientific documentation no one can dispute the existence of vertebral subluxation. This documentation is available through the University of Colorado in their annual publication of our research efforts at a cost of $15 per issue.

"The human body is not perfect. I know about practically every chiropractic theory and I know a great deal about spinal biomechanics –and still I have occasional problems. There is no doubt that the environment acts as a stress to the body. Especially where there are weak areas of problems previously uncorrected. The body has a difficult time coping. So we get symptoms and will continue to. Patients should be checked for VSC on an ongoing basis. In essence, I do recommend chiropractic health care for practically everybody...

"VSC changes the entire health of the body. This has been proven many times. The spine is not an isolated structure. It is an integral part of the central nervous system. It is a dynamic living organ. It can almost be said that it houses a 'brain'...yet, it is like having a brain in your spine. What then can be more important than the spine. We have proved that VSC causes not only structural dysfunction of the spine and adjacent tissues but it also causes nerve dysfunction."

Other important research

In the developing appreciation of research that is now evident within the chiropractic profession, an example is a recently published comment of Scott Haldeman, MD, DC, PhD, who stated, "Research that I consider valid indicates that spinal manipulation is as effective or more effective than other treatment modalities for certain acute and chronic spinal pain syndromes, as well as referred syndromes such as cervical, brachial, and dorsal neuralgias and sciatica, and a variety of headaches."

44

College developments

In a March, 1983 issue of WORLD-WIDE REPORT, Marjorie Johnson, DC, Director of Research administration at Palmer College of Chiropractic, in Davenport, Iowa, brought the profession up to date on the part being played by the chiropractic colleges in the area of research:

"Chiropractic research is a responsible answer to chiropractic practitioner, faculty member, student, and patient need. Such research contributes to the growth of the body of knowledge in the health sciences, in general, and the profession, in particular. And in essence, realistically, serves an overall humanitarian purpose.

"Chiropractic colleges have, subsequently, been the sector of the profession challenged to provide the logical locus for scientifically structured chiropractic research activity.

"The mandate to the colleges is clearly appropriate; –the tasks proffered, handleable (but awesome in magnitude) to say the least.

"Palmer College of Chiropractic, responding to the rapid expansion of chiropractic research possibilities, moved to a decentralized research systems approach in mid-1981. In so-doing, Palmer joined ranks, in a manner of speaking, with an increasing number of colleges and universities in the US reporting non-centrally administered research programs.

"The Palmer program is continuing to pass successfully through successively more complex phases of campus research sophistication as regards research projects. A marshalling of college resources is accomplishing goals.

"The innovative change in Palmer research administration was initiated to more fully realize Palmer faculty creative research talents and capabilities. Each academic department is responsible for meaningful research projects within its faculty.

"Palmer College is recognizing that the entire college community 'must contribute to the research effort.'"

Initial osteopathic research

From a 1982 report from the Kirksville College of Osteopathic Medicine Press, by J S Denslow, DO, it can be seen that this profession, too, has had their problems in getting under way with research. It is reported that "The first consultant was Dr George H Steinhaus...a physiologist of national stature with a particular interest in what, today, would be called 'wellness' or 'physical fitness'." Basic biological mechanisms, it was decided, were to be researched.

Research was started in what was then the new field of electromyography.

Here, now, is an observation from the osteopathic profession that could even help to explain what has been elaborated on, early in this text, under the heading of "Principles" as they, initially, incorporated the idea of "tone."

At the time of the initiating osteopathic research, according to this report, it was thought, and taught, that the resiliency --the so-called "tone"--of skeletal muscle was due to a rotational contraction of small groups of muscle fibers even though the muscle was at rest. However, Dr Edmund Jacobsen, a psychiatrist at the University of Chicago, used EMG to demonstrate that "normal" skeletal muscle action potentials are present. He also observed that in certain psychiatric problems, muscle contraction was occurring. This he attributed to what he called "reflex tension." He developed a therapeutic approach to certain psychiatric disorders which he called "Progressive Relaxation."

Interestingly, phenomena that were discovered are now being used, clinically, as "biofeedback" techniques in physical medicine and rehabilitation.

The osteopathic profession is very enthusiastic toward research developments within their profession and are appreciative of the progress of the profession as a consequence of entering into extensive research projects.

Chapter IV

UPDATING

Need for proper terms

Doctors (whether DCs, DOs, or MDs) are, sometimes, slow to change over from older terms in use during a period when they were related to values and understanding of that outdated period with knowledge not yet advanced, further.

Terms become antiquated, with a failure to discard them and replace them with words that fit more into the understanding of the newer times.

Dr Karl Menninger, at one time, called attention of a conference of colleges to the matter of failure to use proper terms. This was a conference titled "Exploding Frontiers of Science" and attended by representatives of the business world such as IBM and others, and institutes of higher learning such as Barnard, Bryn Mawr, Mt Holyoke, Radcliffe, Smith, Vassar and Wellesley.

Dr Menninger cautioned his audience in the use of words: "Such terms as psychopathic, psychotic and schizophrenic are little more than high class Greek profanity and have no business in the vocabulary when it comes to describing the mentally ill."

Dr Menninger said, at the time, he had used such terms 40 years previous to this period but added that increased scientific knowledge and more complex methods of dealing with mentally ill had antiquated the terms. That same thought, of course, can be applied to the vocabulary changes that are needed in the chiropractic profession to bring it up to date and in the terminology used to convey ideas to the public to, also, bring them up to date.

Words discredited in the mental health terminology of twenty years ago are not used as extensively, today, but are

47

still kept alive and in vogue by those who are slow to discard them.

Dehumanizing terms

It is not just the chiropractic profession that has need to watch use of terms. At the 1984 annual meeting of the California Medical Association, physicians were advised to avoid such terms as "provider," "consumer," "vender," and "gatekeeper." They were warned that these are terms of marketing origin that dehumanize the physician-patient relationship.

Nomenclature for chiropractic

Over the years, there has been an encouragement toward chiropractic science to establish a vocabulary of its own.

Medicine, it has been declared, employs a medical terminology to express strictly medical thought. And it has been claimed the chiropractic concept, as a clear and understandable presentation, is not conveyed well with medical terminology.

Use of medical terms by the chiropractic physician in the presence of those accepting the medical concept causes confusion and uncertainty.

If it is necessary to present the chiropractic concept in medical language, the only gain would be in the providing of an opportunity to go further into the subject and use the instance in order to explain just what is meant by adding the chiropractic interpretation.

Insurance influence

The insurance industry made extensive inroads upon the vocabulary of chiropractic when it became necessary for the profession to either use the terminology of medicine in diagnostically describing what it is the chiropractor concludes about cases under care or substituting strictly chiropractic terms and educating the insurance industry to their use. The tendency has been to cater to insurance programing with medical terms.

At one time, for insurance purposes, there was an attempt to substitute the designation "Vertebrogenic Somatic Dysfunction" for the chiropractic spinal subluxation. It never became universal in acceptance.

In some instances, there is, presently, an attempt to substitute the non-specific "manipulation" term for the chiropractly applicable "adjustment." And though many words have been written in protest against the adoption of the less significant term of manipulation as compared to the recognized and understood chiropractic adjustment, there still persists an unintelligible use of this manipulative term as an intended substitute for chiropractic adjustment.

In the case of "manipulation," it is not a matter of replacing a term with one that would be an improvement. It would be replacing a term with one that does not convey the specific incorporation of a basic chiropractic procedure.

A comment from the book, "Guide to Chiropractic Management (Paul Smallie, DC)," states "Tradition, habit and usage of words have influenced man in the consideration of his state of health." The book suggested chiropractic wording, in a diagnostic sense, to help to more realistically deliver chiropractic conclusions for insurance purposes. The terminology was presented under the heading of "non-pathologic diagnosis." But due to extensive controversy over the use or non-use of chiropractic diagnosis as an accepted part of chiropractic procedure, at the time, it seems   nothing developed from this suggestion.

With that thought in mind, the book was revised and republished in 1980 under the title "Chiropractic Diagnosis."

The first three opening paragraphs of the book read:

Due to general public acceptance of commonly-used disease terms, chiropractic physicians find themselves faced with the necessity to deal with the application of an identifying of terms for non-existent disease-entities as they proceed to administer care after making some form of identification of the functional process that is in need of their particular attention.

The greatest influence upon the chiropractic profession, of course, in the matter of requirement for classifying and labeling variations in the state of general health, has been the insurance industry.

Since it is impossible to classify disorders merely by referring to the area of nerve involvement interference, --mainly, since this fails to show the degree to which the body is responding in its effort to recover--, the need has been for use of a strictly chiropractic form of identification. But the tendency is to provide medically-oriented insurance reports with medically-oriented language.

Truth in words

How do you describe what you have discovered in connection with your patient's health? Just tell the truth, in your own words. And, above all, be honest!

Surprisingly, many words are dishonest within their meaning with the thoughts they convey.

Using the word disease in the sense of arousing fear with its use is dishonest. Implying words like virus include a meaning of attack to produce disease remains a very questionable meaning.

Even the words health and sickness can carry with them a degree of vagueness, with a need for more specific explanation.

Health might be more honestly described as a condition of the tissues of the body providing one with an awareness of comfort as these tissues respond to environmental influences.

Words relating to health will carry a more honest and intelligent meaning when the world becomes more aware of the chiropractic approach to health matters free from unacceptable medical concepts.

Scientific mind and facts

It is unfortunate that research is sometimes undertaken, primarily, for the purpose of supporting or verifying, to the satisfaction of the public, some theory which may have no acceptable basis except an illogical arrangement or misarrangement of demonstrable facts.

The scientific mind is willing to approach any subject in question -and then accept that which stands the tests of truth, irrespective of its nature or where, how or by whom discovered.

Truth and science

Truth is that which may be accurately expressed in terms of unqualified correctness as to any fact or facts.

Conclusions may be true, but it must be possible to give expression to such conclusions along with the logic by which they are reached.

Science is truth. The scientist is one who has knowledge of truth as it may be involved in, or a part of, a particular science. And only truth can serve as the basis for science.

Logic

Logic is the means of distinguishing truth from that which is false, even if it deals in conjecture.

Logic is the means of establishing harmonious relationships of alleged facts in the process of arriving at correct conclusions.

To be a science, there must be a sustaining by logic or physical demonstration.

In the chiropractic profession, great attention has been given to the importance of logic in the scientific considerations dealing with conclusions arrived at in determining chiropractic concepts.

51

No one would contest the importance of the use of logic, however, this does not cover the full reasoning process when arriving at determinations simply on the basis of logical consideration. Before one can enter into logical considerations, there is the matter of perception. Everyone experiences a variation in perception, depending on previous, personal experiences. Perception, of course, is how we see a situation, --how we conceive it to be, in the first place, before applying logic. To start off with biased perception, for example, there can certainly not be anticipated an objectively logical conclusion. So the argument favoring logic does not hold true unless there is objective, unbiased perception to begin with.

Word interpretation

Everyone knows the difference between a noun and a verb.

In a sense, the big controversy over the difference between the medical concept and the chiropractic concept, in regard to use of the term "disease," adds up to whether we consider the term as representing an object, --which would make it a noun, or whether it is primarily an action, --which would make it a verb.

If disease is a noun, then it is a thing, --an entity. If disease is a verb, then it is an activity, a malfunctioning.

An example can be found in the world of psychology. Would you call a thought a noun, - a thing--, --a something statical? Or, would you call it a verb, - because it is dynamic in action and does not remain still but continues on as an activity, or function. In fact, if you stop to think of it, you will see that thought can never be a noun because no thought remains stationary as though it were a thing to be examined in a standing-still state. (This is why it is difficult to scientifically examine thought.)
A thought is an ongoing activity, and the moment it registers as a thought, it continues on into the next stage of thinking. So when you are dealing with thought, --you are really dealing with thinking, - in a sense of movement. And this applies to,

and even helps to explain the clouded controversy in regard to disease, - one of the biggest areas of disagreement between the medical and chiropractic professions.

Disease is not really a noun for it is not a term that represents something that exists, separately, within itself (...although described as such by the medical profession). And this is where the chiropractic concept more honestly pictures disease when describing such as a malfunctioning activity taking place as part of bodily activity or, as it is sometimes referred to, –as "pathophysiology."

Sickness is a reaction causing awareness of discomfort in response to environmental influences. The degree and extent of functional impairment would be in relation to the consequent discomfort.

False theories and false dramatization in relation to health matters are dangerous. And, today, such are responsible for much of the current state of ill health.

Facts

Presumptive facts result from hypothetical reasoning upon a mixture of certain intangibles and tangibles occurring in mental processes in reaction to some known and some unknown stimuli. Alleged facts should be presented along with a statement of reasons and logic upon which they are based. This provides a complete honesty of presentation and assurance of complete understanding.

In chiropractic considerations, there need be no quibbling over the nature of energy. The fact of energy is generally accepted in science.

There are many manifestations of energy influence. Among them are a consideration of the various rays that seem to be more or less universal and in constant motion.

Though not all being perceptible to the senses, these energy rays may be influential in the orderly processes that characterize space and its contents.

Electricity is one manifestation of energy generally accepted as fact. Its transmissibility is also accepted. And recognized are the effects upon organized and unorganized matter, --both in the process of organization and disorganization.

In the light of the many discoveries in energy research, it would seem logical that all organized matter may come about by condensation and retention of bombarding energy rates.

Chapter V

EDUCATIONAL ASPECTS

Openness

There should be no thought of trying to monopolize knowledge gained from the study of chiropractic science. Science facts are for mankind. They should be made available for the advancement of humanitarian causes.

Principles

The educated doctor is a person with an extensive knowledge of the principles by which living processes are influenced. A knowledge of these principles prepares one for outlining the program for influencing living processes of protoplasm, consistent with the conditions of the environment. Skill in making intelligent environmental adaptations comes from knowledge of principles and experience in applying them.

The chiropractic physician should consider every factor by which living processes may be influenced. The education is in relation to every aspect of health. The properly educated chiropractic physician is a general practitioner.

Education in the chiropractic profession has been described as incorporating a knowledge of principles. Techniques and skills constitute the arts of application of the principles.

Anyone understanding a principle is in position to employ his or her own reasoning power, logical and honest thinking, to develop the necessary skill required under the varied facets of learned experiences.

Knowing of gravity, one then has to proceed to necessary adaptations in a world influenced in its entirety by gravity. There is an openness, here, for this to either have a satisfactory or unsatisfactory influence. This would depend on the accuracy of calculations made, and the good or bad of it is only natural.

Gravity, magnetism, affinity or whatever one chooses to designate, is the force that causes all combinations of matter (both living and non-living), all of which have attractive power characteristics of each.

It is by cellular processes that living continues. All cellular processes are either/or a combination of mechanical, chemical or thermal influences, varying with the specific attractive powers of the different substances entering into these processes.

Qualifications

The chiropractic profession should remain vigilant and protect the public from those who would pretend to engage in chiropractic practice without the necessary qualifications. The MD for one, is not properly qualified until so-educated.

Texts

There is great need for expanding the number of texts related to all subjects required in the study of chiropractic science. There is also a need for surveillance to help to ward off literature that is authored in a manner that disregards the ultimate effect upon humanity if such literary creations are not supported by facts.

Scientific knowledge

The chiropractic student has been fortunate in being exposed to a chiropractic education that helps the future doctor to use his/her faculties of judgement based on scientific knowledge and a conditioned pattern of thinking that encourages the doctor to depend on his/her inner understanding that has been absorbed during academic and clinical exposure during the educational process.

That which is presented in textbooks foreign to chiropractic conclusions should be seriously weighed in the light of the extent to which chiropractic education may supercede that of authors outside the sphere of chiropractic education.

56

Every facet of chemistry and all other subjects required are in perfect harmony with the principles of chiropractic and if correctly analyzed provide -by logic and the rules of reasoning- an indestructible foundation for the doctor to successfully maintain his/her po sition in the scientific world.

Chemistry

One should know enough of the laws of chemistry to know the absurdity and impossibility of making an accurate test of any of the circulating fluids of the body. In fact, it should be known that cellular and fluid chemistry is in constant process of change and cannot be determined as of any particular time.

The chemistry of the living human body, being constantly in a state of flux, is unknown and unknowable.

One of the most wonderful facts imaginable is the ability of the human body to regulate its chemistry, fluid pressure and temperature throughout life.

Functioning and adaptation

Knowledge of the automaticity involved in functioning and adaptation to perpetual environmental changes should be a prerequisite to chiropractic understanding.

Scientific principles

The purpose of concerned attention to chiropractic principles is to afford the chiropractic student an opportunity to apply the scientific principles found only in the correct presentation of known facts of anatomy, function, and biological processes for maintenance of cell-life in the human body.

Dr T F Ratledge, during his lifetime, never stopped impressing upon the chiropractic profession and its areas of educational institutions the importance of recognizing that chiropractic knowledge is consistent with science. He constantly reaffirmed the fact that chiropractic is not in conflict with science in any respect.

Biological science

Due to the historical controversy that has attended the chiropractic effort of the past in the area of pioneering to introduce a newer concept into the world of health education, it would be most important to recognize that chiropractic education is consistent with the facts of science, -specifically, biological science.

If all doubt can be erased from the mind of the chiropracticly educated doctor, it allows such graduate to go out into the world of health service with the highest respect for his/her professional fellowman and for his/her own self-esteem. And with that vibrant enthusiasm inspired by knowledge and understanding in a self-assured manner, along with a certainty toward personal ability to apply the principles of chiropractic science, the graduate is prepared.

Self sustaining activity

Chiropractic should not let itself, as a profession, be restrained through wasted effort in engaging in comparative debate with those whose indoctrination prevents their openness to considering chiropractic approaches to health matters. We are not in a race with medicine and can stand upon the merits of what can be demonstrated from chiropractic education.

Prerequisites

It would be of advantage for those among chiropractic educational faculties to be so well versed and thoroughly indoctrinated with an understanding of chiropractic that there would be openness to freely explain, meticulously, an adhering to chiropractic principles and the chiropractic premise which includes every manifestation of the living human body, whether associated with health or sickness.

One should know sufficient chemistry to explain why the introduction of chemicals into the human body, when derived from sources other than air, water and food are considered to be foreign and dangerous to health and life.

History and research

In the history of development of chiropractic as a science, unheard-of benefits in general health matters were, initially, sufficient to arouse the curiosity of those who contacted chiropractic procedures closely enough to get the trend of the basic reasoning underlying the practice.

With extensive research into the subjects of anatomy, especially of the nerve structures, secretory and muscular cells –and of course the connective tissues which form the framework and general supporting structures–, the individual and associated functioning, it will be found that sufficient evidence exists to proceed along chiropractic lines of investiagion and conclusions.

Although chemistry is a science, it cannot be applied, scientifically, except under circumstances where every element to be combined is known. In the world of commerce and industry, chemistry is definitely a science.

In the form of a chemical, every medicine or drug is coming from manufacturers, doctors and pharmacists who know the chemical composition and purposes for which they are intended. However, since the chemistry of body fluids is unknown and unknowable at any given time, the administering of drugs ceases to be an exact science. Such administration becomes distorted even from constant changes from respiratory contributions, exhalations from gaseous products of metabolism for instance, and similar ongoing physiological events.

Irregularity of dependability also enters into the commonly referred to "side-effects." In this instance, there is an apology for injury due to the use of known chemicals used with good intentions, of course, yet without knowledge of the chemistry of the internal environment of the human body.

59

Chiropractic science addresses itself to the human body and its function, --not to what diseases are thought to do as a primary entity to be dealt with, directly.

All recovery from injury depends upon cellular metabolism. And no chemical introduced into the body is helpful unless it is derived from ingested and digested food and/or water or air.

Lower animals consume only that which is indicated by the senses, i. e., food when hungry, thirst when the body requires more water, and an increase in respiration when more oxygen is necessary.

The special mechanisms that function within man are so-constructed and constituted to correctly provide for his physical needs.

Every symptom of so-called disease is the manifestation of the body reacting to the environment. And it is the exclusive responsibility of the body to regulate and maintain the internal environment. It does this through functional activity of the structures that extend to every cell of the body.

Excessive stimulation from the environmental consistency (either mechanical, chemical or thermal in nature) excites contraction in muscles, and since a great majority of muscles are related to --and parallel to the spine-- they exert a great influence on the nerve system by producing such compression on the intervertebral cartilages. These become thinned and permit obstructive pressure on nerve trunks, thus impairing essential functioning. This is automatic and unavoidable. It will result in retention of heat, retention of fluid with proportionate swelling and redness due to dilation of blood vessels. Altogether it presents the typical condition known as inflammation.

Educationally, the nerve system received very little consideration until chiropractic discovered the influence in matters of health.

The psychological and psychiatric aspects of sickness are very important and, automatically, become a factor in all professional care of the sick.

Psychological benefits

Confidence of a patient in the alleged effectiveness of any corrective effort, or confidence in the educational background of the doctor - and in the doctor, himself-, takes the burden of responsibility from the patient, resulting in muscular relaxation and freeing of nerves from obstructive pressures, with corresponding improvement of functioning and maintenance of a neutral internal environment.

This factor, although often overlooked, is highly important and automatically becomes involved –irrespective of the doctor or type of service administered.

The patient gets well on his own power. The doctor –or the remedy– gets the credit.

Physiology

Dr T F Ratledge, in his lifetime, insisted that physiology, as presented at that time, and generally accepted, was written exclusively in support of the medical theory, showing how physiology of the human body is affected by diseases. This form of education, maintained Dr Ratledge, is not suited to chiropractic instruction since chiropractic science considers that satisfactory health is only possible with adequate and coordinated functioning of the entire body.

Chiropractic educational institutions, insisted Dr Ratledge, should abandon efforts to blend medical and chiropractic theories.

Public education

As an obligation in the interest of the public, it should be the duty of chiropractic physicians, in organized actions, to help to expose that which is practiced in a manner detrimental to the health of the public.

The people, for example, have no way, on their own, to find out the injury to which they are subjected, accepting in child-like faith the toxic chemicals from drug administration that can confound the functioning activities within the natural manifesting of life of the human body.

Chiropractic is a science and cannot afford to continue the use of unscientific language in its discussion within the profession or in its use in presentations to the public.

There is a huge public out there, --both in this country and throughout the world--, waiting for the scientific message of chiropractic to be delivered in understandable language.

Chapter VI

CELLULAR RELEVANCY

Importance of cellular knowledge

Under the heading of fundamentals with which the chiropractic physician is concerned is the consideration of the trillions of body cells that make up the human. They are specified as functional and non-functional. A most important consideration in the total of life and health matters is the importance of the functional cells.

Resting upon these functional cells is the entire responsibility for the maintenance of a normal cellular environment within the body and /or adaptation to influences arising outside the body. And this continued responsibility can be met only by continued adequate functioning. It is at this point that chiropractic science has interjected itself into a consideration of actual cellular health in order to establish a platform of understanding.

The consideration of the activity of the human functioning cells is a study of the world, or the universe, within itself. Facts from such study are of primary importance. And the chiropractic student is engaged in concern for the basic knowledge rendered from examining such facts.

Life within the cells

Many uncertain theories of life, per se, have been expressed, and the idea of life being a principle of universal extent seems more logical and specific than any of the several interpretations.

Some believe that life is a specific force. Some believe that nerve energy is the specific life force. So far, there has been no material device, or plan, for proof of any of the various suggestions.

63

The "universal principle" would seem the more preferable version which would make life automatically and perpetually available to all cells and associate the materials in proper amounts and combination for metabolism. This, of course, is the process by which all cells live, dependent as they are on a satisfactory environment.

In connection with life within the cells, there are certain basics to be considered, here:

(1) The sole effect of nerve impulse to a cell is stimulation.
(2) Nerve energy is a transmissible energy. It is generated in the nerve cell body. And with the possible exception of the recording of nerve cells of conscious centers is projected over nerve fibers to other cells which the impulse stimulates, causing them to function.
(3) The cells of the human body, as stated, are the functional and non-functional.
(4) The functional cells are of three types (previously listed): nerve, muscle, gland.
(5) Non-functional cells are classed as connective tissue cells. They serve as the framework for the body structure and all of its organs.

It is important to establish this.

Function

Cells are "functional" and "non-functional."

The functional cells, doing all the work, are comparable to the movable, or moving, parts of machinery. Non-functional cells make up the framework, being classified as "connective tissue" cells. These include the white fibrous tissues, cartilage, ligaments, tendons, aponeuroses, septa, membranous covering and lining of all internal organs and body cavities, lungs, tubular structures, bronchial tubes, blood vessels, etc.

The functional cells of the human body are of three distinct types. They are nerve, muscle and gland cells. The nerve cells are the most numerous and most widely distributed.

All functional cells must be stimulated to manifest character-istic activity of their respective types.

Stimulation implies the chemical process occurring in the po-tential energy producing chemical substances previously ex-tracted by cells from food, water and air, and stored in the cell together with the thermal and mechanical changes occur-ing during stimulation.

All stimulants are either mechanical, chemical or thermal in nature. And they arise, respectively, from chemistry, pressure, tension and temperature of the environment. This factor will be referred to, repeatedly, for it is an item of major import-ance in any consideration dealing with the responsibility in health variations.

All matter has the quality of chemical composition, density and temperature. And it is important to note that the cells of the body have individual tolerance to the three natural quali-ties of the human environment. Changes in these initiate stimulation. The intensity will determine the degree of funct-ional response. This is very important.

All of this is important in relation to the ultimate creative ac-tivity with which the doctor is constantly dealing in consider-ing degrees of health.

No type of non-functional cell can be stimulated. The only action taking place within them is that of metabolism in its de-structive or constructive stages. And this, of course, is com-mon to all cells.

A consideration of metabolism is basic. It is the process of living and of death of the body. Life continues upon both phases of metabolism. When the constructive phase of meta-bolism stops, this is really the end of life.

Cessation of respiration has been accepted as the time of death. But this can only be an arbitrary designation. Respirat-ory activity has been known to resume after respiration ceases.

A well nourished functional cell contains sufficient chemicals from which to produce the energy for customary periods of work to which it is adapted. Work of sufficient intensity or duration results in fatigue of functional cells in varying degrees. This is determined by the depletion of energy producing substances failing to be replenished.

Extreme degrees of fatigue are labeled exhaustion. Recovery from this state of exhaustion is experienced with (a) a lessening or cessation of the work load along with adequate availability of food, water, air and(b) a satisfactory environmental state, along with (c) a period of time to allow food to be eaten, digested, absorbed and distributed. And this distiribution, of course, is accomplished by circulation of fluids to the cells that involves chemical affinity, attracting all chemicals needed.

Nerve cells must be stimulated to produce energy essential to functioning. And no functional cell is stimulated unless subjected to direct effects of an irritant. To re-emphasize: Such irritants may be one of three types: Mechanical, chemical or thermal.

Mechanical, chemical or thermal qualities correspond with the qualities of all inter-related matter. And it is this inter-relationship that accounts for the spark of life that keeps it all in operation.

If the matter of the environment presents enough difference in quality compared to that of the cell substance, it will then result in combustion and the production or release of energy essential to cellular functioning.

Irritants, or stimuli, are classified as primary or secondary. And, again, they may be mechanical, chemical or thermal in nature.

If these irritants are primary, they arise -exclusively- from environmental influence.

Secondary stimuli are produced, exclusively, from nerve cells. The product is known as nerve energy or nerve impulses. And the next major step for the chiropractor to be aware of is that if there is no obstruction from pressure on the nerve cell axone, then the impulse remains transmissible and is transmitted on to intermediary cells (These are nerve cells) in the neural arc involved. And the nerve impulses may also be transmitted on to either muscle or gland cells.

It is assumed that some of all three categories of cells participate in any coordinated body-structure functioning. And to further elaborate, it should be added that there is no evidence of either category of functional cells being involved, alone.

Since primary stimuli arise in or from the cellular environment the first cells affected are the sensory cells which are the beginning of the neural arc. These usually terminate in relation with muscle or gland cells. (There is an exception, here: The exception is to terminations with intermediate nerve cells in ganglia, external to the brain, --or in relation with nerve cells within and constituting the memory areas of the brain.)

The term function is more appropriately reserved for changes in cells occuring in response to application of stimuli in the interior, or surface, of functional cells. Much new material in the nature of cell surface sensitivity has been recently generated with the extensive use of computerized and electromicroscopic procedures constantly yielding newer information.

These chemical changes --which should not be thought of as just in relation to the process of metabolism-- take place in such functioning cells in the release of energy, when stimulated.

Energy, so-released, causes contraction, a shortening and thickening of muscle cells, or lessening in diameter of gland cells. And it is through this means that their secretions are expelled, or for sufficient rigidity of nerve cell bodies --where they serve as chambers from which the nerve impulses are projected into the axones through which they are transmitted to other functional cells where they, mechanically, stimulate the

the cells to which they are distributed.

The functional cells do all the work within and of the body, including movement of parts. Such activity, on a more massive scale, ultimately becomes even ambulation of the body, itself. It is the functional cells that are responsible for the peristalsis of the tubular structures in the movement of air, water and food as this material is distributed throughout the entire body.

As far as life is concerned, each cell represents a world within itself. The essential provision, of course, being that it must have a suitable environment.

Blood cells are a transient type of cell and they are not part of the fixed tissue cells of the body. They have no power of locomotion and are pushed along in the circulating fluids of the body. This takes place in the blood and lymph channels through which the neccessary body-use-elements are distributed to the fixed tissue cells. This, as well, incorporates the area from which degenerative and waste products of catabolism are removed from the internal environment of the body.

Red blood cells ordinarily appear to be non-nucleated. But when circulating through the capillaries where they come within range of the chemical affinity of the tissue cells, they lose sufficient oxyhemaglobin. They lose their color and are then classed as white corpuscles in which the nucleus of the corpuscle becomes visible.

Leucocytes are elderly and deteriorated red blood cells, or victims of serious earlier injury and, correspondigly, defective.

Each cell is a living unit and re uires substances derived from food, water and air to maintain itself in the living state --to remain alive.

Cellular activity

A cyclic periodicity seems to be approximately 24 hours for balancing the constructive and destructive phases of metabolism, the uninterrupted regularity of which is essential to health.

During the constructive phase of metabolism, the cell acquires chemicals from the intra-somatic fluids, blood and lymph. These are built up into potential energy and protoplasm of functional cells - or in non-functional cells- restoring normal chemistry and cell protoplasm.

If cellular metabolism is not balanced within the normal cyclic period, degeneration or sickness begins and fluctuates with environmental conditions.

The general body environment includes everything, or condition, which exerts any influence upon the body. Therefore, in order to make more easily understood this process, we divide the environment into internal and external.

As the name implies, the internal environment is the interior of the body, inclusive of the cells and the fluids, blood, lymph and secretions. It also includes the various systems, --the contents of the air passages of the respiratory system, the alimentary tract and the reproductive and urinary systems.

The external environment includes everything outside the body, as has been stated. And it includes that which is not regulated by the functioning of the body structures but relates to that which may exert any influence upon it. For example, this includes sun rays, cosmic rays, x-rays, etc. These serve as illustrations of external environmental influences, some of which do - more or less continuously-- affect the body, while others occur only occasionally -either by accident or intent.

And now, coming down to the relationship of the cells in the general economy and makeup of the human body, the human body structure is, exclusively, made up of cells. It is important that this be kept constantly in mind as a means to simplify any consideration of the human body and its function.

Makeup

How many cells constitute the human body is unknown and unknowable. Extravagant guesses have been made by the professionals. But your guess is equally good.

All cells have a common structural pattern. Although globular, they become variously shaped as they adapt to stress of growth.

Most cells have a nucleus. And this primitive organic matter is, as we know, called protoplasm.

It is at once apparent that the number of body cells is astronomical and cannot be, intelligently and practically, studied and analyzed except by classification and separate and associated consideration. This must be given to each class of cell.

To accomplish the high volume of activity that must be accomplished to process and distribute nutritive substances throughout the entire body and move the body in space, certain specialized cells must conduct this activity (functional cells) while others play a passive part (non-functional).

Nerve cells most numerous and most important (as stated), play the important role of making possible the coordination of functional activity throughout the entire body.

To simplify the mechanics involved in functional operation, it can be stated that the functional cells require a stimulus that triggers the release of energy by the cell to which the stimulus is applied. The same substance, circumstance, or condition that may act as a stimulus to a functional cell will only precipitate chemical degeneration --or catabolism-- in a non-functional cell. This degenerative phase of metabolism is considered from a medical standpoint as disease.

When both constructive and destructive metabolism are equal throughout the entire body, it is in perfect health. This means that the functional response to environmental stimuli is proportional and adequate.

Nerve cells are divided into two groups that we are all familiar with. They are sensory and intermediate.

Sensory nerve cells are numerous and so widely distributed

that it may be correctly stated that they are found wherever need for functional response to an environmental unneutrality exists.

These are the general points that need to be stressed at this time and will be dealt with in less generalized form later on.

A knowledge of these basic facts prepares one for the simplification of the more complex problems with which one regularly deals.

Summarizing

To sum up, there are six main points to be considered:

(1) Atom cracking has been the chief means of generating or releasing, to the extent of cellular needs and consistent with the potential protoplasmic stress of the cell, ever since the first one was organized. To illustrate logical evidence of cellular ability to generate a vast amount of energy from very little organized matter, this is the difference between the amount of food consumed to meet the daily energy requirements of a healthy working male and the amount of energy that could be produced from the same amount of food if artificially processed.

(2) In general, the manifestations of energy in the human body may be for purposes of consideration, arranged into two categories, the direction of energy-travel to be the determining factor. One category includes the centripetal or magnetic types of force manifestations. The other category comprises the centrifugal manifestations and is the only type of energy manifestation subject to specific, voluntary or conscious acts which may be employed to influence the energies of the body.

(3) Magnetic energies are entirely responsible for all metabolism and all chemical changes in the cellular protoplasm and in the fluids of the body, whether such change be constructive or assimilative or destructive.

71

(4) Centrifugal energy is responsible for the excitation of the processes of stimulation in all coordinated cellular functioning.

(5) Cells are grouped into two categories and designated as functional and non-functional. Functional cells are those which may react to stimuli or to some particular intensity of stimulatory influences. Non-functional cells are those of which the entire framework of the human body is formed and merely give form to the body and to the organs, and providing the necessary rigidity and flexibility to the various parts of the body and contained organs. Non-functional cells cannot be stimulated or caused to do work any more than the wall of a house would be made to work by electricity wired to a motor installed in the floor of a basement.

(6) All cells of the human body live by the same means and similarly die. The term metabolism includes all chemical processes in living cells including both constructive and disintegrative phases which simultaneously occur in varying degrees in the individual from the time of union of male and female components until such time as all chemical change in the cell is degenerative, –at which time only does living cease and death prevail in the cell.

Self regulation

A careful observance and analysis of living animals and plants of the world strongly indicate the great influence of environment upon the characteristics of each. One can take, for instance, the difference between marine plants and those found on land. Similar species in different climates or atmospheres and altitudes show marked variations in adaptation to extreme temperatures, atmospheric and fluid pressures. Also, wide variations are seen in plants and animals of the humid swamps and those of arid areas.

Life, in its variations and complexities, becomes a fascinating study in the unveiling of its simplicity of makeup, –all readily

72

available to indepth study through concern for the vastness of knowledge potentially packed within the living cell.

Osteopathic commentary

The cell is full of "organelles" that carry out many functions. Even the cell membrane is a living, functioning structure. And only part of its purpose is to contain the cells' inner makeup states the May 1977 issue of the JOURNAL of AOA. It refers to an "adapted" cell as differentiated from a "diseased" cell and describes the adapted cell as one "capable of performing its appropriate function(s)," whereas the diseased cell is either unable to perform these functions or does so only with harm to itself. And it adds, "we can stay health only by maintaining homeostasis and much of this homeostasis maintained by our cells."

Using hypertrophy as an example, the article author observes that hypertrophy is not always pathologic but may merely be a highly successful adaptation and the involved cell, at worst, an adapted rather than a diseased cell.

Research recommendations

Along chiropractic lines of reasoning, it has been asserted that each organism has an endogenous, goal-seeking mechanism for sorting, integrating and acting upon psycho-physico-chemical information from internal/external environments. Psycho-physico-chemical processes (or what T F Ratledge would have called "mechanical-chemical-thermal influences") enter into this physiological goal-seeking that incorporates a direct/indirect link between body cells.

Etiological relations between body cell and neurophysiological phenomena continue to be explored. And in the area of nutrition, there is research into the consideration that axoplasmic transfer and conveyance may be the mechanism providing long term maintenance of specialized cells.

73

Radioactive materials applied to selected nerve-cell bodies were shown to be conveyed through the nerve path, across myoneural junctions into the muscle tissues. In studies, axonal components transferred to muscle were found to be protein, and it was found that protein delivery occurs in this manner in four distinct waves: The first, at 6 hours; the fourth, 30-35 days later.

So it has been suggested that chiropractic research is also aware of neurotrophic factor involvement.

It has only been in more recent years that a more wholehearted concern has been evident in the fact that trophic function is not limited just to motor nerves but is also being considered in the activity of sensory nerves. This is an area that has been and is gaining necessary attention.

Indepth cellular study becomes particularly important when there is the realization that the full answer is not supplied from clinical research, alone. Chiropractic cannot limit its research to its unique methodology. There must be investigation at the cellular level as well as the clinical.

If cortical control is a factor, then this should be incorporated as a potential governing center for cell activities. Chiropractic and experimental cell biology as a unit of investigation –in such considerations as cellular surface sensitivity– could be an area of enlightenment for the scientific community. A possibility of this nature was proposed by Cyril D Anderson, PhD, of Texas Chiropractic College, in 1975. The observations immediately preliminary to this are from Dr Anderson, as well.

Dr Anderson has suggested that "if events responsible for total regulation of normal cell processes can be correlated into one unified model, causes can then be traceable to imbalances in cell regulation." "If necessary," concludes Dr Anderson, "specific secondary factors contributing to aberrant function can be identified, later."

Chapter VII

ENVIRONMENTAL INFLUENCES

Recognition

An important distinguishing feature in the presentation of chiropractic concepts by T F Ratledge, during his long period as a recognized and respected educator, was his profound differentiating in the matter of consideration of the recognition of the inter relationship of the human --in matters of health-- to the environment.

This has been a most overlooked area due, probably, to the influence of BJ Palmer's philosophical presentations that tended to limit concern to the brain and its innate intelligence as the starting point for all mental and physiological activity.

It has been the influence of the insistence of T F Ratledge and others that we go back beyond this point and recognize what happens before the brain, itself, goes into action with its accumulation of innate wisdom.

To say that the innate intelligence, about which so much has been written in chiropractic literature, must originate in the brain is to deny the additional demonstration that each cell includes signs covering this innate intelligence in considering matters of health; the full story is overlooked unless this admission that all living cells manifest such innate intelligence is included in conclusions related to the subject.

Regardless of any inherent or external force coming into play as an instigating factor --where ill health is concerned--, recovery is still dependent upon restoration of satisfactory nerve coordination and delivery for proper functioning.

This area of imperative concern, when scientifically considering all aspects of neurological functioning of the human body, has been, sadly, neglected. And because of its neglect, chiropractic has been criticized by the scientific community in failing to deal with the full scope of application of chiropractic principles as they truly exist and function in relation to every activity associated with the life and health of the human body.

Non-philosophical

T F Ratledge did not accept the philosophical view that you could just completely disregard all environmental influences in considering the health of the human body. It was his studied conclusion that if you had something that was outgoing from the brain, downward and then outward, you also had to have something, correspondingly, coming inward that you needed to deal with as well as considering that which was expressing itself in a downward and outward manner, within the body.

T F Ratledge directed attention to a dealing with the degrees to which the body reacted to influences from both the internal and external environment, thus, providing knowledge of a full and complete consideration of all influences that relate to the degrees of health and functioning of the human body.

T F Ratledge, in his directing of attention to the subject of the body and its relation to the environment, taught that satisfactory health is an automatic and inevitable result of adequate functioning control of the environment, ---internal and/or external.

Functional control

Functional control is dependent upon adequate production and distribution of nerve energy. This must be delivered to the functional cells in all parts of a complete, unsurgerized and living body. And this human body would, necessarily exist in an environment so constituted that the related tissues would be able to adequately respond to every degree of unneutrality arising in its environment (internal and/or external).

The varying degrees of departure from a neutral environment are of prime importance in realizing the development of the original causes of health variations.

Types

Primarily, the environment presents itself as mechanical, chemical or thermal factors, occurring either externally or internally.

To come back, for a moment, to what has been stated as BJ Palmer philosophy regarding where "life force" originates (as he stated it, "from above, downward"), it should be stressed, here, that a distinction has to be made wherein it should be recognized that in one instance we were talking about something philosophical and, in the other instance, something scientific. We should avoid confusing philosophy with science. They can be interrelated, but they are separate.

BJ Palmer

The BJ Palmer reference was philosophical and did not refer to "nerve activity" but to "life force" (in the philosophical sense). So we should be cautious not to infer that there can be comparison, - one with the other. One, it is repeated, was in the philosophical sense. One was in the scientific sense. Both can be acceptable without cancelling out the other.

In the non-philosophical sense, it should be stated that all nerve energy or nerve impulses do not have their start in the brain. They are generated in all nerve cells --indluding the peripheral, sensory cells and all of the intermediate nerve cells situated in the numerous ganglia.

Taking these factors into consideration stems from a concern for the scientific consideration.

Interjecting the philosophical is something apart from the scientific. And while it may have its place, an updating of philosophical reasoning should be in the sense of interpreting scientific facts.

To call nerve energy "life force," does not necessarily negate the philosophical concept.

77

Stimuli influence

In accordance with the intensity of the stimuli and the ability of cellular reaction, all functional cells will react according to classification, i. e., nerve, muscle or gland.

Since muscles contract, gland cells also contract and discharge their secretions, and nerve cells integrate and project impulses of nerve energy when stimulated. And since the spinal muscles run parallel to the bones and intervertebral cartilaginous discs of the vertebral column, the contraction of these muscles tend to pull the vertebrae. To the extent vertebrae are thus approximated, the openings, through which the spinal nerve trunks extend, become smaller, and if enough, may cause obstructive degrees of pressure on the nerves lying in the involved joint.

Degree

The exact degree to which obstructive pressure begins is unknown, but there is a definite maximum that may be determined by future research --of nerve pressure consistent with tolerances-- which, no doubt, vary with the quantity and density of the connective tissue sheaths which surround the axones of which the nerve trunks are composed.

Nerve energy and force

Nerve energy arises out of the catabolic processes in nerve cells situated in lower centers in the spinal cord and nerve ganglia (as well as in the nerve cells of the brain), and in either afferent pathways.

Gravity, magnetism, affinity or whatever one chooses to designate, is the force that causes all combinations of matter (both living and non-living), all of which have attractive power characteristics of each.

Nerve interference

Obstructive pressure on nerves is, first of all, bodily defenses against violence from the environment, whether mechanical, chemical or thermal.

The first conscious reaction to excessive stimuli is muscular contraction and heightened fluid pressure upon the nerve fibers and dendrites in the soft tissues to obstruct (to some extent) the transmission of impulses during the period of heightened pressure and, correspondingly, minimizing discomfort or pain from the excessive stimuli. As general pressure is reduced and the nerve response reaches the center of consciousness, the individual consciously lessens the degree of contraction, gradually, --which results in minimizing discomfort or pain or shock that would otherwise be experienced.

In the general contraction of muscles, it should also be noted that the spinal muscles contract and, momentarily, --or as long as excessive stimuli are applied--, exert obstructive pressure upon spinal nerves by drawing the vertebrae closer together, and thus lessen the diameter of the openings in which the spinal nerves lie.

As soon as the stimulus is sufficiently diminished, there is corresponding relaxation of the muscles and the intervertebral vertebrae apart and to their normal distance from each other. Thus, automatically and inevitable, the nerves are freed from obstructive pressure at the spine. If, however, the nature and degree of the injury prolongs the period of contraction and compression of the intervertebral cartilages, they become more or less fixed in their diminished thickness, and cannot expand to separate the vertebrae as they did when not subjected to long periods of compression.

Putting the patient to bed is medically considered a means of conserving the energies of the patient to better resist the disease. Actually, putting one to bed permits muscular relaxation, expansions of the intervertebral discs, enlargement of the intervertebral foramina, freeing nerves of degrees of obstructive pressure on nerves and so, proportionately permitting an in-

79

crease in transmission of nerve energy with resulting functioning, and of course, the neutralizing of the internal environment and corresponding improvement in health.

The patient's recovery depends upon his own nerve energy, and putting him to bed increases his access to that energy.

Concluding, it is important for every chiropractor to be aware of the interdependence of man and his environemnt and to appreciate how the material qualities of man and his environment so inter-related as to influence and affect the ongoing health factor variations to which man is subjected at all times.

It is through knowledge of these inter-relationships that one can readily perceive how health disturbances can come about and how they can be helped, both in a benefitting sense and in the sense of prevention.

Chapter VIII

PHYSIOLOGICAL CONCEPTS

Primary considerations

Since it is the process of cellular and body functioning that is responsible for maintaining a satisfactory internal environment, this becomes a primary consideration in dealing with health problems.

Environment and sensitivity

The quality of one's environment, --either internal or external and the state of one's sensorium are what determine the nature or intensity of functional reactions.

An unneutral internal environment is neutralized either mechanically, chemically or thermally. This is done through functioning.

All substance is of chemical composition and attracts substances to itself as a result of magnetic forces in relation to their affinity. Cells live by acquiring substances through their own power.

In changing substances, the processes that materialize are thought of as metabolism. The whole process of metabolism is merely the process of combining and separating of substances under varying forces.

Metabolism is an automatic chemical process that occurs in the cell in accordance with chemical laws, just as definitely and dependently as it would in any laboratory, depending on what chemicals might be combined.

Metabolism is the means by which cells live.

Function is the result of stimulation, and stimulation is the result of stimuli. And these are the result of differences occurring between environment and the body itself.

Stimuli occurring, first, are referred to as primary stimuli, --occurring, first, are referred to as primary stimuli, --occurring just with change in environment.

After our sensory cells are stimulated, we have a secondary stimulus.

Nerve energy is a stimulus. It has no other value. It results in the functioning of the cell or cells to which it is transmitted.

Next to be considered is the activity associated with blood corpuscles:

Blood corpuscles can be no more normal in serving the body than the qualities of the internal environment will permit.

The combined chemicals of which corpuscles are composed, apparently, provide the magnetic quality by which they attract oxygen from the inhaled air in the lungs.

On the return trip from the tissues of the body to the lungs, they convey gaseous waste to be discharged into the air to be exhaled.

Growth and development of blood corpuscles are dependent upon the qualities the internal environment will permit. These qualities are the three qualities of matter, --mechancial, chemical, thermal. All are satisfactory only to the degree that functioning is adequate to regulate internal environmental qualities. These qualities are regulated by functioning of the three types of functional or working cells.

The reason that functional cells become inadequate in functioning is the fact that they cannot function without energy. This energy is -or shouod be- coordinated and associated by the nerve system.

Nerve cells react first to primary stimuli, --mechanical, chemical, thermal-, arising from the environment. Nerve energy is essential to all functioning upon which environment maintenance depends. The health of the corpuscles is no better than the environment to which they are related.

There is no doubt that the energies of the body are all of an electrical nature and produced in each functional cell for the needs of that cell. These cells are nerve cells, muscular cells and glandular cells.

Nerve energy is a transmissible energy. It becomes a stimulus suited for normal and coordinated operation of all functional cells of the body.

The human body may be likened to a plant in which all machinery units are electrically motivated, but none of which will operate without receiving a proper amount of nerve energy.

Maintaining a satisfactory internal environment is the responsibility of functioning.

Satisfactory maintenance of the internal environment of the body is entirely dependent upon the functioning and coordination of the nerve, muscular and glandular cells.

From the moment of fertilization of the ovum and/or spermatazoa, and during the entire span of life, metabolism is the sole process responsible for the characteristic changes in cells, down to complete disintegration after death.

Injury to cells precipitates degenerative change, and only as the effects of injury are overcome by reestablishment of coordinated functioning and restoration of neutrality is restoration of cellular normality possible.

Considering the subject of physiology strictly from the light of chiropractic interpretation, it can be disclosed that some conclusions are, naturally, at variance with medical conclusions.

There is an apparent general agreement among anatomists that the human body is made up of, variously guessed at, trillions of cells. Each of these is responsible and empowered by nature for the processes necessary to life and continued living.

There are just two general classifications of cells, --as has been stated, before- one of which forms the framework of the body and includes the bones, ligaments, tendons, cartilages and soft connective cell tissues. The other class includes all of the working, or functional cells. These are nerve, muscular and glandular or secretory.

All functioning or activity within the body starts at the sensory nerve cell which is stimulated either by chemicals, temperature or mechanical stresses of the environment.

Our environment includes everything that has any influence upon our bodies - even the sun is in our environment. Environmental influences can be classified under the headings with which readers are now very familiar: mechanical, chemical or thermal. Importantly, these are the sole factors of all cell excitation or functioning.

The sole function of muscle cells is contraction.

When muscle cells are stimulated, an automatic response to contact with some stimulus causes catabolic changes in the cell chemistry which produces muscular energy that then excites contraction or a shortening of the cell fiber.

Functioning of a nerve cell is similar to that of a muscle cell except that the catabolic changes set up in its chemistry results in the production of nerve energy which is projected from the cell body over a nerve fiber, --or axone--, one of which every nerve cell possesses (extending to other cells, other nerve cells, muscle cells or gland cells, which are proportionately stimulated with the intensity of the impulse of nerve energy).

84

Stimulation and release of energy in a cell is imperative in proportion to the energy producing chemicals, or potential energy, stored in the cell.

Recovery from injury is due, exclusively, to external forces and to the powers of the body as manifested in constructive and destructive metabolic processes.

Cell structure, classification and physiological potentials, must be known in order that the science of chiropractic can be understood.

The spine

Discovery by D D Palmer of irregularities in human spines, followed by their apparent coincidence with illness, led to efforts to adjust vertebrae which, if successful, brought about improvement in the health state. Then, the next logical step was to find out why. This led to study and research concerning vertebrae and associated structures.

The uniform existence of notches in the upper and lower lateral borders of each vertebra, forming the intervertebral foramina, occupied by spinal nerve trunks (each two vertebral bodies being united by an elastic disc, forming a sort of universal rocking-joint which permits limited flexion of the vertebral column in any direction with corresponding decrease in size of the foramina) forced the conclusion that varying degrees of pressure on the foraminal contents would disturb physiological, or functional, activity of the contained nerve and vascular structures with which they were associated.

Since nerve trunks transmit impulses of nerve energy and supply stimuli of great speeds to all of the functional cells, by which function is coordinated, it was concluded that such pressure as would reduce the transmission of nerve energy was the most important consideration in the matter of any variation in vertebral relationship.

The question of reduction of the diameter of blood and

85

lymph spaces or vessels in the foramina was not important because of the frequent branching. Collateral channels would suffice.

So vertebral adjusting is commonly used as the means of correcting obstructive pressure upon nerves for the purpose of re-establishing normal transmission of the high-speed energy and coordinating stimulus for any or all of the functional cells of the body.

The exact degree at which obstructive pressure begins is unknown, but there is a definite maximum that may be determined by future research of nerve pressure consistent with tolerance which, no doubt, varies with the quantity and density of the connective tissue sheaths which surround the axones of which the trunks are comprised.

The chiropractor who does not know the purpose of reducing obstructive pressure on nerves is not applying chiropractic principles and is not practicing as a chiropractor.

In the consideration of physiological processes, one should bear in mind that all primary stimuli arise from the environment (either internal or external) and are the result of mechanical, chemical or thermal variations in the environmental substance, to such intensities that their prolonged continuance would injure the tissues through fatigue. Later, through inevitable and natural degenerative metabolism of cells.

Muscular tensions are the immediate and inevitable result of any degree of excessive stimulatory qualities occurring in the environment, either internal or external.

The first --or immediate-- tensions are protective, causing pressure on nerves to obstruct sensory, or afferent, impulses and prevent painful intensities of nerve impulses from reaching the area of the brain where consciousness occurs. Simultaneously, intervertebral cartilages become compressed, permitting the approximation of contiguous vertebrae and obstructive degrees of pressure on such nerves as are distributed.

86

Congestion

In relating physiological processes to ill-health, one can consider the matter of congestion in the various structures of the body. This may occur in any of the tubular structures, arteries, arterioles, and capillaries, venules, veins and the heart, itself, --thus reducing the supply of oxygen, and removal of carbon and other catabolic by-products, and removal of other degenerative chemical elements which must be eliminated from the body. By the same token, the heat produced by oxydization to some degree in all cells of the human body, is not conveyed to the ordinary points of escape from the body, increasing the temperature and manifesting in so-called fever.

Under such impairment of functioning in the vascular system (blood and lymph) such rise in temperature is imperative. And it is equally imperative that the temperature is proportionately reduced with the increased rate at which the heated fluids arrive at the portals of heat exit from the body.

The skin and lungs are the principle avenues of heat escape, but the heat must be brought to them before escape is possible.

Sustained (chronic) impairment of functioning and exposure of the cells in any tissue of the body to retained irritants, --whether mechanical, chemical or thermal--, undermines cellular vitality and, depending upon the time of exposure and the intensity of the irritants, cells may reach any degree of degeneration and will manifest, accordingly.

From the primary changes in the cellular protoplasm, not visible to the unaided eye, to the first perceptible dilatation of superficial blood vessels through the walls of which the color of the contained blood makes the surface more or less red, as in mild superficial inflammation, to varying stages of cellular degeneration before complete death of the cell occurs.

Degeneration, functionally

To illustrate the fact of various degrees of cellular degeneration, the degree of degeneration which is erroneously designated cancer (as a disease entity), or that of gangrene (or of complete necrosis of cells), the only difference in any of such manifestations is degree of degeneration in the involved cells.

All evidences of degeneration in cells, irrespective of degree, are primarily due to the failure of the body to function adequately in the task of maintaining a satisfactory environment for its cell-health.

Restore normal functioning and health is imperative except where vitality has been permitted to get too low.

Psychological involvement

Obstructive pressure on nerves is, first of all, bodily defense against violence from the environment. The first conscious reaction to excessive stimuli is muscular contraction and heightened fluid pressure throughout the entire body, thus producing enough pressure upon the nerve fibers and dendrites in the soft tissues to obstruct to some extent, the transmission of impulses during the period of heightened pressure and, correspondingly, minimizing discomfort or pain from the excessive stimuli. Of course, as general pressure is reduced and the nerve response reaches the center of consciousness, the individual consciously lessens the degree of contraction, gradually, and this results in minimizing the discomfort or pain or shock that would, otherwise, be experienced.

In the general contraction of muscles mentioned, earlier, it should be noted that the spinal muscles contract and, momentarily, exert obstructive pressure upon spinal nerves by drawing the vertebrae closer together and thus lessening the diameter of the openings in which the spinal nerves lie. This, of course, would be contingent upon the duration of application of excessive stimuli.

As soon as the stimulus is sufficiently diminished, there is corresponding relaxation of the muscles, and the intervertebral cartilages, being elastic, reexpand and force the approximated vertebrae apart and to their normal distance from each other, thus, automatically, and inevitably, freeing the nerves from nerve pressure at the spine.

Should the nature and degree of the injury prolong the peri-od of contraction and compression of the intervertebral cartil-ages, they become more or less fixed in their diminished thickness and cannot expand to separate the vertebrae as they originally did when not subjected to long periods of compression.

Physiological factors

The physiological story of the body is screamed at one when considering its structure. This means tissue classification, cellu-lar arrangement and functions and the facts of environment and its influence upon health.

The completeness of chiropractic is surely clear when analyz-ing the body and the corollary of secondary principles har-monious and in no way conflicting with the basic principle of chiropractic science.

In the matter of cellular considerations as related to physiol-ogy, each cell must attract from the blood and lymph any and all nutrient material that may be utilized.

Blood cells live just as do all other cells. But they have special affinity for oxygen and are very fragile.

Being continuously moved through the lungs, the blood cells acquire oxygen proportionate to their magnetic powers.

Fixed tissue cells are far more powerful in structure and mag-netism. Therefore, they exert a stronger pull on the oxygen in the passing corpuscles. They take oxygen from them proport-ionate to the needs of the fixed tissue cells. With this oxygen in the corpuscles, there is enough to influence the color, caus-ing a taking on of a red color, –but not as red as corpuscles in the arterial blood in the systemic arteries, aorta and its branch--es.

89

All corpuscles are primarily white, becoming red only when carrying a sufficient volume of oxygen.

The characteristic presence of white corposcules in the blood is due to the presence of corpuscles which have been denuded of oxygen by the excessive oxidation in actively functioning cells or in areas of congestion in which there is always diminished oxygen supply.

When the oxygen-laden red corpuscles reach the capillaries, the tissue cells of the area extract --through chemical affinity magnetic force-- the oxygen. Accordingly, they then lose their color. If the demand for oxygen is great enough, they become white corpuscles, --as has been stated and restated for emphasis.

Red corpuscles serve as oxygen carriers to the fixed tissue cells. In areas of impaired circulation, the oxygen supply is deficient, proportionately. This results in increased loss of oxygen so that the corpuscles become white (as been stated to help visualize this more thoroughly). There is then loss of vitality and degeneration, losing hemoglobin and ceasing combining with oxygen, through the lungs.

Adequate oxygen supply to the fixed tissue cells of the body is the most important factor of all influences in the maintenance of health and life. Any impairment of circulation correspondingly reduces the oxygen supply of the tissues of the involved area, resulting in a corresponding degree of cellular degeneration (medically considered pathology). Such degeneration is natural and imperative when circulation is impaired.

When tissue cells become devitalized to the extent that they cannot be revitalized and restored to a condition of health, but do not die, medical conclusions state that a chronic disease has not only attacked but has decided to remain and coexist with its victim.

Local injury such as cuts, bruises or burns block circulatory channels, causing retention of fluids, congestion, marked dilation of blood and lymph vessels, increased stimulation and combustion with characteristic heat production, swelling and elevated temperature (medically termed fever).

Blood cells are as capable as any other cells in adapting to changes in the environment. In other words, they may become low on their magnetic power and attract less oxygen and undergo degenerative change, even to the point of death in case of sufficient injury from an unneutral environment. But they may be restored if the environment is restored to a tolerable degree of variation in unneutrality.

If the environment is sufficiently tolerable for cellular rest, all cells may (if not specially injured to too great degree) become fully restored to satisfactory, or normal state of health. This is presupposing there has been no degree of injury too great to allow recovery.

Just as functional cells used in voluntary activities require adequate periods of rest, so must the non-functional cells have rest periods sufficient to reacquire the chemicals lost by oxidation under the stresses of unneutralities resulting from undesirable temperatures, chemicals and mechanical factors occurring in the environment.

Nutrition

None of the above mentioned restorative processes can take place without food in a proper state for cell use. This proper state of nutrient material cannot be attained except by proper digestion.

All foods are good when properly digested. Otherwise, all improperly digested foods irritate and injure all of the cells of the body. So it appears that the matter of digestion is far more important than the kind –or nutritive potentials-- of food.

Digestion

Digestion of food is definitely a chemical process. And there are chemicals that will mix with certain chemicals but not with others.

All chemical processes, irrespective of how simple or how complex, require certain specific periods of time for completion.

Testing food

No test (chemical or otherwise) of food --any foods-- will, if made prior to its being subjected to the digestive process, guarantee its being proper for any individual. The degree of value of food cannot be determined unless tested after digestion is completed. Even if such a test could be made of substances in the alimentary tract, its value would be doubtful. For digestion in the sense of final preparation for cell use, is not completed in the alimentary tract. In other words, the final chemical influence is not exerted there. For when absorbed into the lymph and carried into the blood vessels, it is acted upon by the oxygen and other chemicals in those fluids. It is known that the blood and lymph contain waste products which may enter into the chemical changes taking place before the food goes through the lungs and is on its way out to all parts of the body in the arterial blood.

Food nutrient values cannot be determined before eating.

Food selection

Eating food --at any time-- is more or less an experiment.

The most accurate way to best determine proper food is through its appeal through the conscious senses, memory, looks, smell and taste. If the selection is proper and we have the ability to digest food, the next hazard is in the matter of time required for completion of the digestive process and the time required for rest of the structures involved in the work of secretion and muscluar effort in moving the substance from place to place as necessary to make the various secretions avail-available in the process at the proper time.

92

Timing

It takes several hours, more or less, depending upon the chemical composition of the food eaten, for processing in the stomach, preparing food for cellular use. Then, assuming correct processing to this point, the now partly processed food is discharged into the duodenum where it acts to stimulate the flow of bile and pancreatic secretions and institutes the next phase of the digestive process.

Digestion is a slow and gradual process in which food is chemically changed in preparation for use by all the cells of the body.

Every stage in such chemical process is very definite and characteristic, though unknown at any stage, as to the time required for any certain degree of progress. It cannot be hurried or artificially modified without modifying, unfavorably, the end result.

To the extent that digestion may be artificially modified, the processed substance is made unsuitable for cellular use.

The term digestion, as used, may mean anything or nothing, depending upon its use in loosely discussing events after eating. The term should be used only when trying to state the completed preparation of nutrient material for metabolism in which protoplasm, potential energy and secretions are built up. From the time of oral processing to assimilation, food substance is in continuous chemical change and characteristic according to the conditions occurring throughout the process.

Just as time is a factor in cooking, it is equally so in the matter of food digestion.

Food combinations

Another important factor influencing digestion and the matter of chemical poisoning from degenerating food in the alimentary tract is the matter of mixing chemically by eating more than one item of food at any meal.

The fool-proof way to minimize or avoid toxic effects from food, spoiled by attempting to combine incompatible items, is to eat only one item of food at any meal.

The temperature, plus time, determines whether food has not been cooked enough, overcooked, burned, or just cooked to death. A cook must know how long to cook any particular item of food. The best food can easily be ruined if the time required for properly cooking it is ignored.

Timing as a factor

It takes approximately all night for healthy functional cells to metabolize properly digested food substances to restore an amount of potential energy equal to the energy used in the preceeding working period. Time is of the essence.

Undoubtedly, the time factor is much greater in restoration of cells in which the process of degeneration has existed for longer periods.

Cases are on record where both motor and sensory paralysis had existed for a period of ten years, the patient in bed, absolutely no nervous or muscular activity in the structures involved, yet those cells show a beginning response to stimuli after about six months of daily adjusting and careful regulation of the feeding, and in eighteen months of similar proceedings in adjusting and feeding there was seemingly restoration equal to the energy production prior to the trouble.

Time is before one. And it should not be wasted. Instead, there should be cooperation with the fact that time will go whether or not one proceeds intelligently and permits the power for good to prevail.

Awareness of needs

The human body is fully and well equipped for accurately indicating through the various sensory mechanisms the chemical needs of the individual.

Surely, a body structure that is sufficiently automatic to sense its needs and (on its own initiative) supply those needs, continuously, for years, deserves the greatest respect. And one's body should demand and receive the full faith in its hereditary superiority and perfection.

Even momentary consideration of life, growth and functioning of the human cells is enough to make known the inadequacies of the human mind in that it can in no way substitute for universal law.

With proper and complete faith in the dependability of the human completeness and adequacy to adapt to reasonable changes in environment, we would never eat except from desires designated as hunger. And then we would eat, reasonably, of the item selected and stop with that.

Having eaten the desired food --or any food-- several hours (8 to 12) should be allowed for digestive processes before eating would be repeated.

Ordinarily, the food desired should be eaten --and alone-- to avoid chemical conflict which is unavoidable when we eat several items of food at one meal.

The stomach --or any other part of the alimentary tract-- is not so constructed that different foods may be placed in different compartments while being digested. And different foods --because of differences-- will not be digested in the same period of time. And, further, the quantity and character of the secretions varies with different foods.

Any cook knows enough to cook some things in a skillet, --some in pots, some in pans--, because they do not all cook at the same rate.

After ingestion of food into the alimentary tract, function is begun with the action of the glands of the mouth, stomach, pancreas, liver and the mucous glands in the membrane lining the digestive tract. This is the muscular activity essential to movement of food when it is finished in the mouth, stomach, duodenum and small intestines, etc.

From the small intestines the substance is absorbed into the lymphatics and then delivered to the blood stream on its way to the lungs where combining with oxygen (one of the most --if not the most-- important chemicals), will be used in the final preparation for cellular use.

Vegetable foods can, when functioning is normal, be eaten twice each day if spaced properly. Meats require more time to digest absorb and be metabolized in the body cells. And if functioning is below par, should not be eaten oftener than once each day.

Fear of food is a great psychological hazard. There is nothing to fear about food except failure to digest it.

Toxic factors

Toxic factors are inevitable when food is not digested. Food, the way it is ordinarily taken into the body is the source of most toxic influence (except for the introduction of medication) with which the human body may be injured.

Toxic food irritates sensory nerve cells with resulting muscular tensions, including the muscles running parallel with the spine, causing approximation of vertebrae and obstructive pressure on nerves.

Depending on the tissues to which the impinged nerves extend will be the particular manifestations resulting from their functional impairment.

Eating

Eat only from humger. Select the item of food that appeals most to your memory of food tastes and/or scents. And, of course, food may or may not look appealing and this, too, becomes a factor.

When the body says no about any food, don't eat it.

Eat only from hunger. This should be a key impression.

Eat reasonably of the food selected.

Do not fear suffering from lack of nutrient substances.

Eat through properly spaced intervals, food carefully select-ed, limited (optimally) to one item at a meal, then allowing proper digesting and rest periods. With such scheduling (especially for those who are ill), the secretions and potential energies become restored and 99% of digestive disturbances are solved.

The completion-time in digestion and necessity to reproduce secretions for next meal's digestion indicate a need for sufficient lapse of time between each meal.

There are 6 to 8 hours involved in responding to the stimuli of food present and in the process of digestion. There must be an expelling of secretions already produced during the prior period of rest following the previously digested meal.

Assuming that it requires several hours for digestion with partial completion in the stomach, itself, food then goes into the duodenum where bile and pancreatic secretions are added. This requires an equal time period for further digestion and absorption to be completed. The next step is a carrying through the lungs where oxygenation occurs. This requires several passages through the lungs before oxygenation is completed. It then passes, repeatedly, through the general capillary system where assimilation occurs before metabolism goes into action. So the point is that with all this there is a definite time factor.

Corresponding time for rest after activity is necessary for all involved functional cells. And it would seem that with such a demand for timing that for optimal considerations during a twenty-four hour period, more than two meals during that time frame places a greater demand on the energies of the body than would be ideal.

Food eaten at breakfast is not available for all purposes until very late in the afternoon –or could even be utilized more the following night in providing energy and chemicals for the next day.

In eating schedules, habit can be a great factor.

It is not recommended that one fast for too long periods, -and then with only one instance for a particular condition.

Fasting is very valuable in some chronic conditions in which the patient has been ill over a long period and the body is filled with retained poisons. But at the end of the fast, great care should be used in beginning a new schedule. The first few times the patient should start with some one item that is really enjoyed as food.

How well the food is digested should be closely observed and judgement exercised in increasing food quantity at a meal.

Although eating should be limited to not more than twice a day (morning and evening), the timing should be just once if the patient is not hungry or does not relish the item of food.

A big consideration is the matter of avoiding overeating. And avoid frequent and multiple items at a meal.

Chapter IX

PSYCHOLOGICAL ASPECTS

New awareness

It was in 1960 that Dr Thomas Szasz introduced the controversial thesis that mental illness is a myth. The debate continues in the world of mental health science, where it is still undetermined, except as a matter of faith, whether or not there is such a thing as mental illness.

Terms like "mental disease," "insanity," are now considered archaic. And "mental illness" is being avoided in the scientific literature.

The chiropractic consideration

In the field of mental health, chiropractic science brings to humanity a new concept of the whole problem, a concept based upon an entirely different premise, and offering the results of years of scientific research into the whys and wherefores of mental aberrations supplemented by effective means of applying the principles from which emanate the chiropractic concept of living and all related manifestations of the human body.

States need institutions for the mentally ill. These should be organized and established as separate institutions where they could have advantages of progress in everything that contributes to human welfare. Many cases now medically considered - or classed- as incurable and therefore hopeless have been restored to society and the joy of normal, free living where they choose, through the intervention of chiropractic care.

First and foremost in importance is the establishing of a chiropractic hospital for chiropractic care of the mentally/emotionally ill. It should be staffed, exclusively, by persons educated in the chiropractic concept and should be independent of any department of state, or any individual, private citizen or public official.

All matters pertaining to the care of patients should be governed by an advisory board of five or seven chiropractors who would organize and elect from its members such officers as best able to serve the various duties.

No person, licensed to practice chiropractic in the state, who practices any alleged therapy or any practice pertaining to the health of human beings that is inconsistent with the chiropractic concept should be eligible for appointment to the advisory board.

Provision should be made for removal of persons from medical institutions to the chiropractic state institution when so desired by parents or guardians.

It should be mandatory to authorize the transfer of any patient from medical to chiropractic institution --and vice versa-- upon receiving written request from parent or guardian.

Mental functioning

It has been agreed that teaching is a science. A teacher must be mentally mature and have sufficient psychological perception to adapt to the requirements of each individual student.

It is generally considered that kindergarten, elementary, and much of high school learning is by imitation.

Some psychologists believe that reason begins after the first experience in which consciousness is initiated.

Every new experience is specifically registered in, or upon, certain cells of the memory areas of the human brain where such registration is permanently filed. All subsequent and similar experiences are channeled to the cells upon which similar registration was, originally, made --thus validing duplication or dual memory.

Every variation in subsequent stimulatory nerve impulses reaching brain cells in the memory areas are, in fact, new experiences and are registered on additional cells of the area, thus adding to the total knowledge of the individual, as of that time.

Experience is any reaction to a stimulus from –or originating in one's environment– which results in new registration or reproduction of memory in response to said stimulus.

Experience in reacting to environmental stimuli established innumerable nerve association patterns between the various cells of the memory areas of the brain through which previous experiences may be considered, as in the process of thought and/or reasoning. The establishment of such associated patterns increase gradually from new experience and from thinking and reasoning upon them, –thus our knowledge is increased. The human brain is the most proficient and efficient organization of matter known to man.

One cannot consider a human and not consider that human's mind. It has an effect upon the individual that is not fully appreciated.

Menninger

Dr Karl Menninger, now 92 years of age, has been quoted earlier in this text. Quoting from Dr Menninger, again, he has said, "Too many doctors are treating their patients as unemotional, unthinking pieces of machinery. The tendency is to assume that sick patients can be treated like automobiles, --passed down an assembly line of specialists and workers for a punch here and wrench there– without the guiding principle of an overall perspective."

Dr Menninger denounced overly scientific diagnosis at a meeting of the American College of Physicians, in San Francisco some years ago. Said Dr Menninger, "Most of the patients that you and I treat day after day cannot be given an accurate, specific, meaningful diagnostic label."

Dr Menninger asserted that a patient's equilibrium may be upset not only throughout   body tissues and body fluids but also by thoughts, feelings, behavior and social relationships.

Dr Menninger said the provocative agent could be a starvation of calcium or a starvation of love.

Psychological factors

Commenting on psychological factors related to health, Dr Henry M Thomas, Jr of Johns Hopkins University, at this same meeting warned the doctors present that "Physicians often fail to appreciate the power that even their lightly spoken words have to instill fear into the minds of patients."

Dr Thomas described how a doctor might enumerate a number of symptoms and then ask if the patient ever experienced these, adding, when told, "No," "Well, you certainly should have some or all of those symptoms with that high blood pressure you have." And so, he remarked, the patient is co-operative and sees to it that she does what the doctor asks by acquiring all these symptoms.

Dr Thomas stated doctors should have "first-hand and intimate knowledge of suggestion, reasoning, persuasion, education, rehabilitation, allaying fear, and the skillful and gentle handling of that most important of all mental attitudes, - hope."

"In many ways," Dr Thomas said, "hope is the best antidote for anxiety."

Direct influences

It has been knowingly stated that the vibrations set up by others affect those with whom they are in contact more than realized. There is a taking on of characteristics of those around one.

A negative person, it is known, can arouse havoc in an organization or a home. When a strong negative personality and a positive personality are pitted one against the other, the negative one frequently becomes the more powerful.

An extremely nervous individual in a position of authority can affect everyone around him/her toward a very nervous state. So the caution has been to have the patient recognize this and guard against placing oneself in position to be unnecessarily influenced in a negative manner.

Indecision

Many a patient is adversely influenced by an inability to make decisions. It can be good advice to patients to be more concerned about making decisions and then acting on them --regardless of whether there is a mistake as a consequence, or not. The important concern is for the emotions that come into play with continued indecision. It can be damaging.

Psychology in practice

In the early 1960s, Dr Goldia B Young, a highly respected chiropractic physician in Oklahoma City, presented a paper to a group of doctors in which she urged an appreciation of the ability of chiropractic doctors to help in the area of mental illness and said:

"There is no valid reason why mental illness cannot be treated like any other illness –in the doctor's office. The main goal is to restore him to the community so that he can function."

"Every single practitioner is, every day of his professional life, utilizing the elements of psychology in the doctor-patient relationship, from the decor of his office to the strong suggestion implanted in the mind of the patient relative to the healing power residing within him or her. A knowledge of the basic psychological principles is a must in the efficient and effective management of every patient, as well as broadening the field of understanding, assistance and counselling...

"Dr W Heath Quiqley revealed that 48 percent of the patients who consult the chiropractor are experiencing a significant emotional or mental disorder.

"We need to seriously consider the chiropractor's role toward mental illness and mental health; otherwise, we shall not be equipped to be, and do, what the enlightened public and governmental agencies expect of the chiropractic profession, or what our own best conscience requires of us, and what our own professional growth and acceptance demand. The study and treatment of man must deal not only with the physical but the mental and spiritual...

"Chiropractic, by virtue of the neurological and physical aid that it can offer the mentally ill, has a logical place in the community health facilities. When chiropractic is included and coordinated with those much needed facilities and services, it can help in the early diagnosis, intensive treatment, long-term care, rehabilitation, and after care of the mentally ill. It can prevent chronicity of mental illness and help in the early return of the patient to society; it often prevents relapses, because chiropractic removes some of the embedded neurological stress which is usually not detected or eliminated by medical psychiatry.

"A wide and costly gap exists in the care that the mentally ill are now receiving, for want of the health contribution that chiropractic can make...

"The prudent and humane mental health authorities, and governmental agencies who are vitally concerned with the problem of mental illness, would uphold and look with favor upon our profession if we would use a greater amount of psycho-therapy in our general practice.

"Let us clear away some of our own misconceptions regarding chiropractic and psychotherapy:

"Chiropractic cannot, and must not be considered as a narrow spinal specialty. By the very nature of our art to the human body, we influence to a greater or less extent the entire body in all its psycho-biological functions.

"We must not overlook that there is a potent psychology inherent in the chiropractic adjusting which is meaningful and effective to the patient.

104

"The psyche of man is not the sole concern of the medical specialists. Psychotherapy is not only a specialty; all governmental health authorities and mental health experts strongly urge members of the healing arts to interest themselves in the mental health problems.

"Our patients often need some psychological aid. Some 40 to 60 percent of our patients have emotional components, along with physical symptoms. For such patients, the chiropractic adjustment is not enough.

" We will continue to progress when we represent chiropractic as a comprehensive science and art of healing, applicable to physical and mental distress.

"All healing professions are increasing their psychological knowledge within the framework of their therapies. Chiropractic must do likewise.

"The student is not likely to take postgraduate studies in psychology if his appetite were not aroused during his college years. It must be taught in the classroom and in the clinic and integrated with the basic concept of chiropractic –then postgraduate courses are useful.

"Chiropractic and psychotherapy are both natural healing procedures.

"The time has also arrived for our profession to become alert and daring enough, to courageously make it publicly known that chiropractic has intrinsic value for emotional disturbances stemming from neurological irritations.

"We can then present chiropractic as a comprehensive, competent, and competitive system of healing, which will put our profession into the advantageous position to demand that our services should also be included in the programs of all those agencies which are planning for the improvement of our communities' mental health facilities."

Chapter X

THE BODY IN ACTION

Recharging

The dream of space scientists has been to invent a self-charging by the rays of the sun. But the functional cells of the human body are all equipped for automatic recharging when in a proper environment. And such recharging is a continuous ongoing event of life.

The involuntary structures that make up the human body function continuously. To accomplish such, this functioning necessitates energy production and consequent activity. There is within this dynamic arrangement a necessary rest period phase as well. It is constituted by an involuntary functioning that is so timed within the cells involved that there will be time to recuperate energy potentials during the short period of rest between each functional activity and the next succeeding one.

Rest and sleep provide the necessary conditions for cessation of voluntary functioning and use of energy. This permits the conservation of potential energy for use during the following period of conscious functional control. It is during the period, also, that the ongoing metabolism of the body is allowed to build up potential energy during such periods of rest from sleep to be used in the bodily economy the following day.

Potential energy that has been stored in the functional cells is derived from a combination of chemicals from consumed air, food and water. The potential energy stored in functional cells is released, activated or kineticised through the anabolic phase of metabolism induced by a stimulus. The by-product of such metabolic process constitutes the main part of waste material that has to be eliminated. This takes the form of gases discharged through the lungs.

The lungs and alimentary tract are the only natural channels for making air, water and food available to the body. But while they remain in these channels they are not available to be utilized as by the cells.

In the matter of air, the element of processing enters into the activity.

Oxygen must be removed from the air in the lungs before it is immediately available to fixed tissue cells for use in the respective stages of metabolism.

The greater part of oxygen taken from the air in the lungs is drawn into the blood corpuscles. This is then distributed to all of the fixed tissues of the body.

It is evident that the fixed tissue cells have stronger affinities for oxygen than the "wandering cells" --blood and lymph corpuscles- from which the fixed tissue cells derive most of the oxygen used by them.

A considerable amount of oxygen taken from inhaled air remains free in the blood plasma and is, thus, also made available to the fixed tissue cells through the distribution of the circulating fluids.

Every activity in life must have a corresponding period of rest. And nature has provided such balance.

Physics

Nothing takes place without a cause. We must have an activating force to produce any manifestation of change or motion in matter.

Chiropractic deals with the laws of matter. First, it deals with an analysis of matter, and through that a practical knowledge of chiropractic, the qualities that are demonstrable in matter and which characterize it are those of density, chemical composition and temperature, --as you know. These become com - mon denominators for all matter, whether living or non-living, whether previously alive or dead, or irrespective of its status.

The human body has to be activated. And the factors entering into initiating such activation are, understandably, important.

The human body does nothing, –nothing takes place in the human body–, except as it arises out of the factors bearing upon matter as stated. There is no stimulus that occurs at any time, anywhere, or in any way, that does not arise out of those qualities or properties of matter. These elements of stimuli are just as certain to occur as it is certain that gravity is effective. And we know that gravity has never ceased to be effective during our lifetime. Gravity has a perpetual influence on the functioning in and of the body.

Man's one big difficulty has been in overcoming gravity. And, of course, he has to know the law in the use of gravity in order to overcome its continuous effects. That is the way he gets his foundation, - because of influence of gravity.

In his power activated mechanization of the body, if it were not for the effectiveness of gravity, man could not get off the ground or, otherwise, modify his position in space. He could not move. He could not go forward or backward.

Internally, the body is forced to offset gravity influence in distribution of substances through its several systems of a tubular nature. And the knowledge of all these factors become an important part of information related to health.

Stimuli production

We now have under observation a universal cause for the incidence of stimuli. This applies to stimuli coming into being or the occurrence of such. And, of course, it is merely the condition of matter, itself, that causes it to have such effect. It is based, first, on the tolerance of one individual, or entity, for the other, –or the substance in one instance as to its cor - responding quality in the other mass of matter.

Environment

The human body must have a certain environment for it to be in a satisfactory state. That satisfactory environment is a satisfactory temperature, a satisfactory chemical composition and a satisfactory density of its environment. If it has those, then it has an opportunity to be all right.

Nothing much has to be done about the environment outside the human body. It pretty well takes care of itself. If not, it is taken care of by the things we devise by means of our nerve system activity.

The nerve system is responsible for all of the comforts we have. The human nerve system is, elementally, responsible for it all. The nerve system and its manifestation, the mind, is the precision instrument that supervises it all. It is that nerve system that supervises every activity of our lives, --from minute to minute, from day to day.

In studying the health of the human body, first of all, it is definitely logical and very reassuring to consider the human body as constituting a living unit with functional powers adequate for maintaining itself in a satisfactory state for whatever period of time may be fixed by the hereditary properties responsible for all individual characteristics of man.

As in the case of all organisms, the human is constituted to carry on the activities necessary to living. And this body is constructed of innumerable protoplasmic organizations called cells. Each is independent to a very appreciable extent in the processes by which all living is manifested.

The process by which a cell lives is termed metabolism. And the essentials of this metabolic process are due to the magnetic characteristics derived, principally, from heredity. These processes are derived, also, to a varying degree, from the stresses of environmental experience.

Every reaction in the human body is perfectly natural for the

109

circumstances under which they are observed.

Is pain unnatural? It is not! It is just as natural for you to suffer as it is for you to be happy.

When the quality of one's environment is sufficiently un-neutral, one suffers, accordingly. The same applies to the internal environment. It is perfectly natural. It couldn't be otherwise.

For continuance of life, suffering is a warning to the individual that something is wrong with that individual's environment.

Internal environment

Coming back to the environment, aside from the environment which we have just discussed, --classified as external--, we also have an internal environment, --each of us, individually. The awareness of its part in restoring health is often overlooked.

The human body, as we know, is composed of a number of living entities called cells. They live in this internal environment as a satisfactory state and keep it that way if there is to be a general overall state of satisfactory health.

Keeping the internal environment in a satisfactory state of health is the responsibility of the body, itself.

Functioning and experience

Chiropractic is particularly concerned with how the body meets its environmental responsibility. It meets that responsibility solely by functioning. Of course there is one qualification to that statement. There must also be an accounting for the instance of existing inherent properties of the cell. The cell, as a living entity, incorporates ancestral experience that will also influence activity.

110

Inherent characteristics are the product of time and experience. Environmental influences constitute experience and have their effect upon living things and their effects become, finally, a permanent quality.

The ability of living things to adapt themselves to a particular condition of environment becomes a permanent, or fixed, quality within itself.

Heredity

The cellular manifesting of experiences can be thought of as being due to heredity. Heredity is a fixation of (or in) matter. It causes characteristic manifestations. And it is a result of time and experience.

Looking at the cells of the human body from the very beginning, it is seen that they have hereditary fixations that determine the range of their adaptive powers. They are the sum total of their ancestral experience which, if you would carry it back a few thousand years, might cover a very wide gamut of experience. But this is what our makeup incorporates. Our responsibility becomes one of maintaining that internal environment in a state satisfactory for our needs. And this can be accomplished only through functioning of the body.

Functional impairment

Functioning is a very important matter for consideration in order to become thoroughly capable in dealing with the problems of health.

Unless one understands how to keep that internal environment in a proper state, then unsatisfactory conditions will develop and health will be affected, accordingly. There is such a thing as accidental injury to the body. And when this does occur, the body, likewise is placed in an unsatisfactory state. And if function is disturbed, sufficiently, death ensues.

Deficiency in functioning results in immediate development of excessive degenerative products of catabolic processes in all

111

of the cells in the involved area, producing increased and continuous chemical, mechanical and thermal irritants until such nerve pressure is corrected.

The second factor, of equal importance, is the exhaustion of the chemicals in the functional cells from which energy is released in the process of stimulation explosion. And having run out of ammunition more shooting functioning is impossible until the stores are replenished.

Obstructive pressure on nerves in the early stages of change from normal or neutral environment (and such change is immediate upon the occasion of inadequate or impaired functioning) is temporarily protective, i. e., in voluntary protective contraction (as in holding the breath when about to receive a blow or other type of injury of which one is conscious). But such contraction must be of short duration or the obstructive nerve pressure resulting from the contraction will impair function and bring about an oxygen deficiency (a very unneutral or poisonous chemistry) in the affected part. Such functional impairment will also permit the retention of the amount of heat produced by increased oxidation in the area, resulting in increased redness and swelling (characteristic of so-called inflammatory conditions), following any type of injury, i. e., mechanical, chemical or thermal, and referred to as acute.

If the functioning in the area remains impaired and unimproved, the condition of ulcer or abscess (depending on location) will develop, –blood and tissue cells destroyed, and pus produced.

If conditions, for any reason, become unsatisfactory in the chemistry, fluid pressure or temperature of the entire internal environment of the body or localized in a limited area and the obstructive nerve pressure that has developed from violent contraction of muscles parallel and attached to the spine, is permitted to continue, the case will continue and grow worse. Such circumstances exist in all alleged chronic diseases. And if not restored, will terminate, fatally. Living or dieing is just a matter of environmental influence and the reaction of the body to such influence.

112

All the degrees between satisfactory states of health and death constitute states or degrees of ill health. Differences that involve varying health states could be stated, more accurately, in terms of degrees.

Cellular influences

Aside from the sensory nerve cells, distributed in great numbers throughout the body and all of its organs and parts, all nerve cells are, intermediately, situated in the nerve pathways of the body. They are there to serve as booster stations and as points of increase in functional association.

After studying the compositon of the body, the next step is an awareness of the necessary arrangement of the cells of the different orders that make it possible for them to do what must be done if the internal environment is to be maintained in a satisfactory state to maintain the process.

The non-functional cells are situated throughout the entire body in such manner as to form a framework of such rigidity --where needed-- that all ordinary movement of the body or of its parts are permitted without injury or interference with functioning.

Non-functional cells are of such character and in such situation that they serve as supporting and connecting media for the functional cells of every order and provide strength for resistance to all ordinary mechanical stresses to which the body --or any of its parts-- may be subjected. This would be by reason of its own functioning or stresses exerted upon it from outside sources.

Where complete rigidity is required, certain cells attract and retain sufficient lime salts -or other calcific or calcareous matter-- to give them the required density and rigidity characteristic of bone. This, as is known, is ossification.

Where less rigidity or greater flexibility is required, there is, correspondingly, less deposit in the fibrous extensions of cells.

In the earliest stages of development, with cellular potentials distinguished in an embryonic mass, there are no identifying characteristics by which any cell may be classified as to type, when mature.

The changes during growth are termed "differentiation." They become sufficiently characteristic for classifying in the various categories of mature cells.

It is believed by some biologists that an embryonic cell may grow into either of several forms of the mature cell classification. This would seem to contradict the known specific influences of heredity and leave no room for selective processes to be brought about by environmental influences.

It would seem more logical that the forces of heredity --which so minutely control color, size, shape, chemical make-up and other characteristics at all other times in the life span (and in which they appear to be rigidly channeled)-- would not lapse into such a brief state or uncertainty at that one particular time in the development period.

The uniformity of physical characteristics in different individuals of a species, when development occurs under uniform environmental stresses, would indicate that the limitations of heredity are imposed in every stage of development.

The existing confusion about the suggested potential electivism at any time in the life period is, apparently, due to erroneous interpretation. This error has to do with observations made at fertilization. There has been much speculation related to successive steps of propagation.

Discussing known arrangement and relationships of cells of the body simplifies the understanding of mature or differentiated cells.It is evident that plants and animals require a continuous supply of certain chemicals in certain combinations for oxygen, nutrition and necessary fluids.

The body is equipped for drinking and eliminating necessary fluids, for eating, digesting, absorbing, distributing and disposing of nutrient material. There are effective provisions for separating nutritive materials from the waste and removal of waste.

The body is also provided with effective means of acquiring oxygen as needed - in amounts required by varying activities. Inhalation and exhalation is imperatively continuous. And it fluctuates with the varying environmental stresses and is imperatively continuous in order to supply necessary oxygen. It is also imperative that the poisonous gases - occuring by transmutation of residual waste matter be removed. These are the wastes from catabolic processes in cells and from oxidation of excess food material that deteriorates in the fluids of the body. Most is expelled through the lungs, and there is the fact that because of this, the lungs become a 'first' as a channel of elimination of poisonous residue from the general metabolism of the body.

The body is like a sponge inasmuch as the cells are so-arranged to provide fluid spaces varying from microscopic dimensions of blood and lymph capillaries. And the cells are so-arranged to form channels of smaller ducts for conveying glandular products to points where they are stored, —or to other points for use outside the glands where they are produced.

To squeeze a sponge, forcing out fluids, there is reduction in the dimensions of the sponge in proportion to the spaces within. If it were possible to similarly compress the human tissues, the proportion of fluid-filled space could be approximately determined. However, the proportion of space is not important since it is safe to assume that there is sufficient for the purposes.

The major item of importance about the spaces is their presence in relation to every cell in the body. The space arrangement makes it possible for every cell to have access to the nutrient material being carried through the capillaries.

115

Fluid movement

The larger channels for fluid movement are the arteries and veins. These are the largest at the heart, but branch, repeatedly, as they extend away from it. They become smaller until terminating in the capillaries that continue to branch and converge to connect with vessels of the opposite side of the blood circulatory system.

Arteries are the channels by which the blood is carried away from the heart to the capillaries. From the capillaries, the blood is carried through the veins to the auricles and on to the heart ventricles.

These involuntary working mechanisms are substantially all tubular. The lymph channels are extensions from the blood channels.

Blood corpuscles may escape from blood channels, producing congestion. This is an important item in accounting for ill-health within the body.

Congestion within the body --as in freeway 'rush hour' traffic- slows the movement of blood corpuscles and decreases the supply of oxygen to the congested area. Because of priority for oxygen, cells then are immediately distressed with slowing of circulation.

Physiological conclusions

Contrary to common belief of physiologists, supply of oxygen to tissues depends more upon the action of the muscles in the vascular walls of local vessels than upon heart action. And these blood vessel muscles are to a great degree independent.

Vascular muscles are wholly independent of heart action in all veins and arteries --except to the extent that the blood started from the heart through the aorta. With the aid of arterial wall muscles, there is mechanical stimulus necessary to excite vascular peristalsis through influence of increased pressure in the area supplied by such artery.

All muscles in vessel walls act only in response to nerve impulses resulting from the stimulatory effect of vascular contents from unneutral factors. These arise either from distention from fluid pressure within the vessels, chemical irritants, or
from distension from fluid pressure with the vessels, chemical
irritants, or from some unusual temperature fluctuation.

Corpuscle color

All corpuscles found in the body are either mature blood corpuscles or embryonic –or immature-- blood cells, the magnetic
qualities of which are not characteristically developed enough
to attract oxygen in sufficient quantities to combine with the
hemoglobin of the corpuscle and thus influence the red color
of the corpuscle.

Changing colors

Red corpuscles detained in a congested area lose oxygen in
proportion to the local need. And many become white –especially where they are pulled through capillary walls into the
slow moving plasma that is in the lymph capillaries surrounding them. This imperative increase of white corpuscles has
been, erroneously, interpreted as an action initiated by the
corpuscle, itself, acting as 'body police.' It is thought of as
having rushed to the scene of such injured and congested
points to defend against the invasion of pathogenic germs, or
viruses. Such white corpuscles are just those unfortunate
enough to be carried by the blood to an area where cells have
stronger affinity for oxygen. And in this instance, the corpuscle loses its oxygen –upon which the red color depends.

Questionable pathology

It is utterly illogical to assume white blood cells remain stat-
ioned in the bone marrow or spleen or anywhere else in the
body. It is just as illogical to assume that, upon injury or alleged invasion (pathogenic germs/viruses), messages to the bone
marrow, spleen, or wherever white corpuscles   be, they will
be sent –ordering the white corpuscles to report to a certain
point in the body and gorge themselves upon any poisonous
waste that may have attacked. Such a senseless theory could
arise only from disregard for the known laws of physics and
sound reasoning.

A germ/virus or chemical mass --any substance seen sur-
rounded by leucocyte protoplasm-- is drawn into it by chemical magnetism.

Limited research

The short life of corpuscles blocks tracing their origin. And
the mitosis and amitosis theory of cell division and reproduction has been so generally confused that research has been limited .

It could be that there is in blood vessel and lymph vessel
walls an embryonic substance that is caused to develop corpuscles as the need for them arises. There are literally billions
of these cells reaching maturity every day. And if it should be
demonstrated that they arise from embryonic substance, they
would have to become detached at maturity.

One conjecture could be that corpuscles, so-changed, are
white during the process of development and before maturity,
and again after that part of their life in which they are capable
of combining with sufficient amounts of oxygen as to make
them the characteristic red blood corpuscle.

Should it be ascertained that such embryonic substance from
which corpuscles are derived is present in the vessel walls, it
might develop that the exhaustion of the embryonic substance
responsible for corpuscular development is the chief cause for
the gradual decline after what we think of as middle life. This
would include progress until the decline in corpuscular production results in their reduction to the point that the body
cannot be supplied with enough oxygen to sustain the living
processes. And death would be the natural result.

Laws of nature

No law of nature is a mistake. Nothing that results from the
fact of such law in operation can be construed as a mistake of
nature.

Living is one manifestation of nature's laws acting through matter. The uniformity of such is demonstrated in the fact that nearly every person having arrived at maturity knows of some action that will 'make him sick' or 'make him nervous and upset.' That knowledge is equally to physics knowledge that led to how to produce nuclear weapons. Nature's laws (laws of physics) are dependable.

If nature's laws were undependable, there would be nothing but uncertainty and chaos in human experience. And sometimes the products of these laws frighten one with uncertainties - (as in nuclear weapons). But disregarding that, there could be no planned existence without a knowledge of inexorable laws that govern our human existence. All man's high accomplishments through science has been due to man's discovery of fragmentary truths of natural laws.

Man's egotism, exceeding his growth in knowledge of nature's laws, leads him beyond the limits of safety within which he is perfectly adapted to environmental variations, leading to what is commonly termed accidental injury or death.

Metabolism

Metabolism is a continuous process. It should not be confused with cell function. Metabolism never ceases. But cellular function varies in proportion to the unneutralities occuring in the environment. Each unneutrality, automatically, presents a stimulus to sensory nerve cells which, if capable of functional response, become stimulated and initiate the successional functioning of the intermediate nerve cells. These are the cells of the neural arc.

The neural arc

It should be recalled that all neural arcs terminate, presumably, in such relationship with nerve cells in the memory areas of the brain, muscle cells and gland cells, of the entire body, upon the arrival of an impulse of nerve energy from the last intermediate nerve cell in the neural arc, - said brain cell recording every phase of functioning (all of which may be consciously reproduced). This includes origin, intensity, association and duration. Muscle cells contract and shorten, and the gland cells contract and expel their secretory products.

Metabolic phase

Unneutrality of the environment, automatic and inevitable, prepipitates the degenerative, or chemically disorganizing phase of metabolism (catabolism) in the cell. This is irrespective of cell type of classification.

Anabolism

A simplified example of what happens is found in the following: A person whose health and functioning are adequate for all purposes is being considered: While sleeping, functional requirements are at a minimum. Degenerative metabolism is at a minimum. Constructive metabolism goes on at a normal rate, varying with the nature and amount of nutrient material then present in the body fluids and, therefore, available to the cells. During this period of sleep the somatic functional cells refine (anabolism) and store substances from which energy for use is made available. This is during the following period of consciousness and increased activity --mental and otherwise.

The threshold of irritability of functional cells is heightened during sleep. Stimulation becomes easier. In due time the individual awakens due to stimulation of cells which, when functioning, participate in the production of consciousness.

With the use of substances from which potential energy is derived, there is a corresponding increase in the consumption of oxygen. There are resulting byproducts which adds to the unneutrality of the fluids of the body and increases the functional demand.

As the period of consciousness continues, the supply of potential energy (acquired during the rest period) becomes less. The threshold of irritability lowers. Greater intensity of stimuli are required to produce energy essential to continued functioning until the individual becomes aware of it as expressed in terms of fatigue. When stimulation becomes more difficult (with increasing fatigue) and a correspondingly lowered threshold of irritability of sensory nerve cells exists, all functional activity is, likewise, lessened, and trouble begins. With properly timed reduction of work demand and with complete rest, the body will be able to neutralize the internal environment. Given time, the body will restore adequate energy material for another day's work. Following this, a similar cycle of rest and restoration will transpire.

The conditions, changes, causes and effects described above are automatic and inevitable in the body. No disease in required to produce them. The automatic restorative processes go into action if and when the environment initiates such. To make a messed up internal environment right, it calls for the re-establishing of adequate functioning, —not destroying the disease.

Injury from within

Although fight or flight are the dominant means to escape danger, one cannot run away from injurious internal conditions. So this leaves fighting.

There is little conscious knowledge of self-defense against the internal environment that produces injury from within.

Where cell structure and placement is concerned, sensitivity is strictly individual. There are no standards to determine how sensitive certain tissues may be. So every dosage of chemicals introduced into the body becomes experimental.

Through irritability, the body is automatically forced to function in self-defense, depending upon its own needs and ability. The internal environment controlling functional cells are the involuntary systems of organs and have no option in functioning when stimulus occurs.

For clarification in better understanding involuntary functioning, all involuntary mechanisms become defensive toward conditions of control in which they are caught up and become responsible.

121

Unneutral environment

To describe what constitutes an unneutral environment, it might be stated that it is the imperative result of the alternations in the periodic activity which supplies the requisite neutralizing elements to the environment and the following period of functional passivity during which oxygen and other chemicals are used and the environment becomes proportionately unneutral. This would then provide the stimulus to initiate yet another cycle of functional activity. So it can be seen that the involuntary functioning is related to the regulation of the internal environment to the needs of the body and thoroughly and dependably automatic.

Nerve energy

Nerve energy is a mechanical stimulus arising in a catabolic phase of metabolism in nerve cells from which it is projected as impulses over their axonic extensions to other nerve cells, muscle cells or secretory cells. Potential energy is released by the process of stimulation in such cell and is confined to the protoplasm of the cell and initiates the characteristic change known as contraction. This is the sole function of muscle and gland cells.

Functioning

Functioning in a nerve cell may be compared to the shooting of a gun. In the gun, there must be some explosive substance to which the substance in a nerve cell (from which kinetic energy is derived) is analogous. In the gun, there must be some device by which the explosion may be timed. Likewise, there must be a device whereby stimulation (explosion) may be timed in order to have coordinated functioning of associated cells. In the gun, the explosive substance erupts with rapid oxidation into the projecting energy. In the cell, the stored substance from nutrients is consumed and transformed into the energy necessary to function.

Stimulation occuring in a nerve cell results in the manifestations of impulses of transmissable energy which –upon arrival at another functional cell– has the effect of a stimulus and may precipitate stimulatory processes in such cell. This, then, in turn, will function according to its kind, assuming that –like the gun-- it is loaded with substances containing potential energy.

Stimulus reactions

The nerve system is precise and accurate in its reactions to every previous and identifiable stimulus ever experienced and recorded in the conscious mechanism. The only guide by which one selects food or drink or refuses food is the nerve reaction of the body as experienced in hunger and thirst.

Intelligent eating comes in timing, work and rest periods and refusing food when the body does not call for food and drinking only to satisfy thirst.

Fluid movement

What becomes of fluid when taken into the body? It is quickly taken up by absorption from the alimentary tract and transferred into the blood stream where it dilutes the blood and waterlogs the blood corpuscles, causing them to swell, –even to the point of bursting. The added fluid increases the work of the heart and all of the circulatory mechanisms, bringing on vascular exhaustion and impairment of the circulation with resulting inflammatory processes that follow congestion and corresponding degrees of natural degeneration. This would be medically termed infection and pathology.

In the physiological approach to the subject of fluid consumption, all degrees of inflammatory manifestations and degeneration are explained and accounted for in a way consistent with laws of physics. These control all physical manifestations in living organisms as well as non-living matter.

Human reaction

The human body may be described as being comparable to an industrial plant where all equipment is electrically operated. Every working unit in such plant must be connected with a major electrical system for electric current. It depends on this force to operate. The operator may switch the current on or off, starting and stopping. If the circuit is broken by a short circuit, this will end function.

When carefully analyzed, every functional reaction of the body is one of nature's protective measures. Every injury is characteristically followed by a corresponding degree of functional failure in circulatory structures in the injured areas. This results in retention of blood and lymph which, under pressure of stronger vascular activity in adjacent uninjured areas, dilates the weakened vessels and fluid spaces in the injured area causing swelling. Distention of the vessels in the injured area makes it easier for the vessels to keep the fluid moving to increase the supply of oxygen and nutrient materials and to remove increased waste matter resulting from degeneration caused by injury.

The weakened vessel in an injured area necessarily moves the fluids more slowly, and thus the increased heat produced by increased degenerative phase of metabolism in the cells of the area cause a local elevation of the termperature, medically called fever.

Dilatation of the more superficial vessels in an injured area causes the red color of the blood to be more visible through the thinned vessel walls, completing the characteristic picture, inevitable after injury of any degree to any area of the body.

Just as heat is used to soften metal for bending, so does nature use moulding and welding broken bones for purposes of adaptation in reuniting ends and edges of broken bones, Soft tissues become more pliable with inflammation and more responsive to adaptative stresses incidental to recovery.

124

Inflammation is imperative and automatic in living tissues following injury in any degree, irrespective of the particular environmental influence responsible for it. And, of course, the environmental influence (you are, once again, reminded) would be either mechanical, chemical or thermal.

All tissues, osseous and less dense, soften under the influence of inflammatory elevation of temperature until broken or cut surfaces reunite by the simple process of fusion.

Research

Medical researchers are just beginning to realize the real significance of human environment and the fact that regulation of the internal environment is almost completely the responsibility of the body. There is no fixed pattern for human environment, internal or external, but the internal environment is almost entirely the responsibility of each individual body. This responsibility is met exclusively by functional and adaptative potentialities of appropriate structures within the body.

Due to research inspired by chiropractic, the nerve substance of the body is rapidly becoming recognized as the principle coordinating factor in all functioning within the body.

In view of all the research into the proposition of energy manifestations and all the uses to which energy manifestation are put, on first thought, it is disappointing to observe that human effort has devised no means for causing controlled energy manifestations (or production) except through the processes of disorganization of matter.

Logical reasoning has led man from his first observations of degenerative or disorganizational processes of decay and combustion - possibly identical except in rate-- through the successive discoveries of how to arrange or condition powder to nuclear fission. Science is now searching for some way to control nuclear energy potentials.

Energy factor

Most important to everyone is the use of energy essential to living. Without this, a satisfactory state of health is impossible.

It is most unfortunate that in general research science the energy factors in the human body have not received consideration commensurate with their overall importance in the matter of life and health.

Researchers in science have seemingly stood in awe of the processes of living and dieing and the fluctuations of health and, seemingly, –without analyzing of the factors involved– have gone along with the ancient superstitions that thrived on mysterious disease powers being more important than the powers of the body, itself, for living. This fundamental error has led to a squandering of billions of dollars in futile attempts to discover something intended for the destruction of what is really a nonentity.

Expanded review

The big key to unlocking the secrets to all life processes is an understanding of unicellular life. Complications that arise in observational interpretation can result from failure to apply the same standards for cellular processes of the body as are applicable for each single cell. Within a billion cells, the life process is the same. To understand the process in one is to understand the process in all.

Cellular organization and maintenance depends on magnetic influences attracting substances, building up into protoplasm that characterizes that particular cell for classification.

As the cell is formed of matter, all inherent properties are subject to all laws that affect or control material processes.

Until some stress of environment modifies or destroys some of the original properties of the cell material, the cell will attract elements in amounts as required to maintain an equilibrum and satisfy affinities created by ordinary rates of metabolism.

All cells are special masses of organized matter but may differ enough to be subject to various classifications, i. e., nerve, gland and muscle cells, in the functional category, and the various connective tissue cells which make up the framework of the body and are in the non-functional category.

The most important difference between functional and non-functional cells is that functional cells have the quality of irritability by reason of which they may be stimulated, while non-functional cells cannot be stimulated. They serve only as connective tissue and constitute the supportive framework of the body. Depending upon the type and arrangment of non-functional cells is the degree of strength and rigidity manifest in any part of the body structure (as in bones, cartilage, ligaments, etc., –or where delicate functional structures, as in nerve centers, blood and lymph capillaries, retina, mucous and serous membranes, etc., are supported).

Metabolism is the process by which living matter is developed and maintained.

The health of a cell depends upon and is consistent with the degree of balance or lack of balance between these phases of the metabolic process in the cell:

1) Anabolism is the result of chemical magnetism and/or electromagnetic forces by which the substances essential to the cellular well-being are literally pulled into the cell mass where they enter into combination with each other to fulfill the needs of a cell of its particular classification.

2) Assimilation is the combining of substances, responding to affinities, after they are within the boundaries of the cell. Within this process they are transformed, synthesized into the cell substance or into refined forms of energy and secretions.

3) Catabolism includes every phase of degeneration of the protoplasm occurring during the life of the cell or degeneration of any of the inclusions occurring in anabolism or assimilation.

127

Under the heading of fundamentals with which the chiropractic physician is concerned is the consideration of the trillions of body cells that make up the human. They are specified -as has already been emphasized-- as functional and non-functional. And this is a most important consideration in the total of life and health matters as they represent the entirety of activity with which a doctor deals.

Resting upon these functional cells is the entire responsibility for the maintenance of a normal cellular environment within the body and/or adaptation to influences arising outside of the body. And this continued responsibility can be met only by continued adequate functioning. It is at this point that chiropractic science has interjected itself into a consideration of actual cellular health.

The consideration of the activity of the human functioning cells is a study of the world, or the universe, within itself. Facts from such study are of primary importance. And the chiropractic student and doctor is engaged in an all-inclusive concern in the consideration of the basic knowledge rendered from such facts.

The facts of cellular activity are found within the study of biology, itself.

Biology, as a study of all animal life, is generally accepted as relating to a discourse presenting a theory of living which should account for every manifestation of living matter at any and all times and under any and all circumstances. Such theory should be universally applicable and should afford logical reasoning as to inherent factors essential to the initiation of living processes, heredity, environment, development, structure, function and the results of satisfactory functioning and functional failure, evidences of adequate or inadequate functioning, decline and death.

Life, philosophically considered as a "universal force," falls into the scientific category of a dealing with its nature in the form of an energy or substance.

While it is common practice to attempt classification of energy or force, there is --in all probability-- only one energy which seems to be universal and is so designated by some scientists. The most acceptable description seems to be that the differences in volume and intensities as they modify matter under differing stresses are mechanical, chemical and thermal.

It is interesting to note that while a cell is living matter it undergoes a constant interchange of substances with its environment and arranging it so that it is transformed into the very living matter of the cell. Correspondingly, the cell returns the waste/degeneration products to the environment and continues the process of metabolism until injury and stress modification prevent a tolerable state of its activity. It is at this time that the moment of cell-death becomes fixed.

A nerve cell or muscle cell produces energy in proportion to the amount of nutrient material used, --far beyond amounts of energy available in the combustion of any fuel in man-made devices or otherwise, artificially.

Assuming an atmosphere near sea level to be most ideal, cells are, automatically, capable of selecting from substances suspended in the circulating fluids any and all substances and amounts of each for which its needs are expressed through natural affinities.

A cell cannot use food until it is prepared through digestion and all undigested food becomes foreign matter, irritating body tissues until every particle is reduced and discharged.

Every undigested particle, absorbed and carried to the lungs, then distributed, becomes an irritant.

No food substance, once absorbed, ever gets back into alimentation. And the lungs become responsible for its elimination. This makes the lungs an organ of prime importance in all functional disturbances.

From here, next comes a look at cellular functioning.

Functioning

Stated briefly, the only function of a muscle cell is contraction. The gland cell also contracts. But the difference in results is the arrangement and direction of shortening of their contractile fibers.

Primarily, muscle cells are either voluntary or involuntary. But many voluntary activities may become involuntary in spite of continued consciousness if and when the primary stimuli is greater than the nerve impulse intensity from activity in the conscious centers of the nerve system.

When muscle cells react due to intense irritants, there is proportionate use of oxygen related to the stimulatory process initiated in the neuro-muscular mechanism. Continued violent nerve and muscular reactions reduce the oxygen content of the fluids and there is developed a distress that can be even a most violent paroxysm of pain from oxygen deficiency.

In the walls of tubular structures, the muscles enter into contraction. This is their purpose for being.

The makeup of the body prepares it to be conditioned to adapt to the stresses of the environment. And the body possesses every device required to control and regulate the status of its internal environment.

Most amazing is the builtin provision that functions to automatically correct effects of reactions to environmental stress.

Chiropractic discoveries

It is good for the practicing chiropractor to be reminded of the contributions to the world of health for which his/her profession is responsible.

Chiropractic science discovered that nerve energy, when coordinated, is the sole cause of all cellular and organic activity essential to life, health and recovery from injury or illness.

Chiropractic science discovered that nerve energy could not be transmitted over nerves when subjected to obstructive degrees of mechanical pressures and that in proportion to the degree of excessive pressure upon a nerve there was an imperative reduction in nerve energy transmitted to the tissues of organs to which the impinged nerves were distributed. Also, it was discovered that in corresponding ratio with the reduced nerve energy to the part, its functioning was reduced, permitting the conditions in which there are injurious stresses exerted upon the parts, causing corresponding degeneration with its train of imperative manifestations.

Chiropractic discovered the builtin provision for, automatically, correcting obstructive nerve pressures in the human body, making it possible for the body to maintain itself in a satisfactory state of health under ordinary stresses and to recover from injury and illness resulting from temporary influences beyond the adaptive powers of the tissues or organs so subjected.

Obstructive pressure upon nerves serves a dual purpose in the body economy. In one instance it is temporarily protective, minimizing the injurious reactions and resulting exhaustion from unneutralities in the environment. In the other instance sustained obstructive pressure on a nerve or nerves beyond a certain non-injurious minimum results in impaired function, accompanied with inflammatory and degenerative processes in the parts so deprived of nerve energy.

Chiropractic discovered that sustained obstructive pressure upon nerves occurs only at points where they lie in an opening formed by notches in contiguous vertebrae, separated by an elastic cushion of cartilage holding the vertebrae apart when the spinal muscles are relaxed and the weight of the body is taken from the spine by occupying a horizontal position.

Chiropractic discovered that nature has builtin provisions for the automatic separation of vertebrae which have been drawn too close together by muscular contraction, or the weight of the body when in an upright position, is in the expansive power of the elastic cartilage which lies between the bodies of the two vertebrae, forming thejoints of the vertebral column.

Chiropractic discovered that nature has builtin provisions for the automatic adjustments of all of the joints of the human spine to the extent that the inter-vertebral cartilages have retained their respective powers of expansion, thus freeing all nerves from obstructive pressure every time an individual sleeps. In other words, if the cartilages retain their normal powers of expansion they remove all nerve pressures 365 times a year, free of charge.

To the extent that nerve pressures are not corrected by the automatic expension of intervertebral cartilages, the chiropractic adjustment then becomes the way by which satisfactory health is accomplished.

A manipulation of the spine does not reach the point of ver-- tebral subluxation –since in the region of such subluxation exists the greatest tension and resulting fixation. A specific adjustment at the point of subluxation is required rather than generalized manipulation.

Chiropractic teaches that unsatisfactory environment is the source of every unneutrality. Environmental unneutralities are, within the maximum of functional control, indispensible for the perpetuation of conditions under which the body may continue to live and remain in satisfactory state of health. Environmental stresses in excess of maximum functional control through bodily reaction are injurious and result in cellular degeneration in exact proportion to stress excesses and their duration.

Heredity and its influence constitutes the first half of the story of living. The other half is constituted in the environment. It may be that environment, over sufficient periods of time, determines and fixes, for a period of many generations, the characteristics of heredity.

Reference to a material world implies subdivision which does not actually exist. Such a basis is unsound for study and research when every phenomenon is the product of universal law. It appears there is one law and one world. And it is impossible to understand any phenomenon without having some knowledge of the oneness of things. To illustrate the thought, chemistry means nothing unless considered in relation to mechanical and thermal manifestations of matter.

Biology means nothing when studied without correlation of the basic principles of life with natural or universal law.

Magnetism

It is obvious that magnetism is a negative force, converging to a magnet where it appears to become modified or decompressed and seems to just become dissipated similar to the force of compressed air after escape from the container in which it was compressed. All matter seems to respond to magnetic force under certain special conditions, or influences. Magnetism is responsible for the constructive phases of metabolism, and it is also responsible for the destructive or degenerative phases of the process. Just as the force of gravity is the cause of the convergence of all organized matter toward the earth, that same force is responsible for movement of matter away from the earth. In other words, everything that goes up is because it was pushed up, or displaced upward by some substance responding to the force of gravity. Even the space surrounding the earth's sphere varies in density because of the diminishing of the effects of the force of gravity as the atmospheric sphere increases in diameter.

Each unity of matter in protoplasm, comprising the cell, is there because of the affinity between it and some element of the cell before its entrance prior to becoming a part of the organized matter of the cell.

Each unit of matter in organized protoplasm can be displaced, through magnetic force outside the cell (having greater affinity than for the extruded substance. And no doubt the latter circumstances predominate in degenerative processes. The violence of mechanical stresses to which wrestlers are repeatedly subjected indicates adaptation to such stresses by both education in muscles and corresponding strength, --adap-

133

tations acquired in training. They seldom have any broken bones, with far less strenuous stresses. There is no immunity from broken bones. There is only adaptative distribution of stress. Through adaptation, one avoids the degree of violence and leverage that would, otherwise, break bones and lacerate the less rigid structures of the body.

Chemical influence

There is no immunity to chemical influences within or upon the body. However, there may be wide differences of tolerance developed.

The fact that certain amounts of certain chemicals are lethal to an average person, that same individual may (gradually increasing non-lethal amounts) develop tolerance for amounts ten times or more, than would have been lethal had it been taken prior to the development of the tolerances stated.

Certain chemicals as strychnine, arsenic, etc., although very poisonous in sufficient quantity, are found in the body. And tolerances can be developed to where considerable quantities may be introduced into the body without immediate or apparent damage. However, any amount, above that available in the air, food and water consumed, is inevitably injurious. The same reasoning applies to all chemicals, --whether classified as poisons, or otherwise.

The intensity-effect of any unneutral factor of the environment may originate in the character of either the chemical composition, density or temperature of the environment, or from the hypersensitiveness of the sensory nerve cells, or of other cells involved in the reaction to a stimulus.

It would be an inescapable conclusion, then, that there is no poison, per se, and that the manifestations observed and generally accepted as being reactions to 'poisons' are, regardless of how violent, protective reactions of the body, proportionate to the intensities of stimuli in an unneutral environment. In the light of the conclusion stated, if classifications as poisons is

134

to be persisted in, there would be mechanical, chemical and thermal poisons.

Mechanical stresses

A good illustration of violent, but more or less coordinated, muscular contraction, would be a wrestler reacting to the mechanical stresses to which his opponent subjected him. The difference between the voluntary resistance to mechanical stress of great intensity and the involvuntary muscular contractions of convulsions from chemical poisons would be that the latter were uncoordinated or unneutralities within the body, exciting sustained, violent and involuntary muscular contractions which (when alternating with periods of relaxation) may be designated as spasm. Also, there are muscular contractions, of every degree which may in part, be due to habit-patterns, −as occurs in so-called epilepsy.

Another illustration of mechanical poisoning would be where shock treatment was being administered and the muscular reaction to the electric current was so violent that bones of the patient were broken. This has been reported.

Freezing or burning would constitute stimuli sufficient to be classified as poisons if the degree of muscular reaction was accepted as the criterion for classification.

Every chemical, in amounts above the point of cellular toleration, will stimulate the sensory cells of the body. Similarly, every mechanical or thermal stress, beyond the point of cellular toleration will stimulate the sensory cells of the body. Each sensory cell of the body is sensitive to all three of the sources of primary stimuli, i. e., chemical composition, density and temperature of the environment.

Cellular functioning

Primary stimuli occur whenever, and if, the chemical qualities, density or temperature of one's environmental makeup varies from a state of neutrality, or passes the limits of cellular

135

adaptation and tolerance. This, of course, is upon the assumption that the cell has sufficient potential energy to respond in functional reaction.

At this juncture it is well to review in one's mind the fact that there are three types of funcitonal cells and three types of stimuli. Of the functional cells one type is classed as sensory. The sensory cells have highly developed qualities of sensitivity and react to every degree of variation from the neutral state of the environment, whether it be a variation in density, chemistry or temperature. The cells of the two other classifications, i. e., muscular and secretory, are not sensitive to ordinary pressures or temperature changes except when they are of extreme intensities.

To illustrate the point, it is only necessary to state that when pressure is direct and of sufficient intensity it causes contraction which, in the muscle cell, shortens the muscle fiber, and, in the gland cell, diminishes the diameter of the cell and expels the secret.ion. Everyone has experienced what is designated as muscle cramping in which the contraction is involuntary and not to be terminated at will. Such muscle cramps may be induced by voluntary and extreme muscular effort, but is self-induced by reason of the great and direct pressure exerted upon each other by the contracting muscle cells, themselves. Secretory cells may be caused to contract by reason of mechanical stress from outside the gland where they are situated. When so-stimulated, they merely expel their secretion without distress, unless there is an inflamed condition of the tissues of the gland, resulting in a corresponding hypersensitivity of the sensory nerve cells of the gland.

The body cells live in an artificial environment for which they are responsible in its maintenance in a suitable state for continuous living. The involuntary functioning in the body, respiratory and circulatory, digestive and eliminative, must, continuously, throughout life, be able to react appropriately to every variation if the body is to be maintained in a state of satisfactory health. Appropriate functional responses are dependent solely upon the nerve system for coordination, without which the environment inevitably becomes unneutral and therefore unsuited for healthy tissues and adequate functioning. A satisfactory environment cannot be established by any means except through adequate and coordinated functioning of a nerve system which is in a state of reasonable energy production and without obstructive pressure upon nerve distribution channels. The introduction of vitamins, food or chemicals in any other form cannot correct a bad internal environment unless the body is able to respond in adequate functioning to the irritating influences resulting from their introduction. It is well to bear in mind, also, that the words irritant and stimulant must irritate, or else it would not excite any action, whatsoever.

It becomes evident, then, that any irritant can be applied in amounts that are equivalent to poison and would excite the same (or similar) degree of injurious reaction (in functioning and in degenerative metabolism) in all cells subjected to its presence.

Nature has provided (where man has not intervened) for a fair balance in changes in matter to such extent that there is provided an adequate check for all energy release. Every use of energy release instituted by man is dangerous except where the laws of release or production and dissipation are known and meticulously observed. Any uncontrolled energy, artificially released, is dangerous and may destroy those who would try to utilize it. Electricity, combustive energy used in our power machinery, airplanes and the energy released from fissionable matter, are examples of uncontrolled energy.

The balance of force in nature is exemplified in the processes essential to the manifestations of life. These processes involve both constructive and destructive phases. In other words, life is the result of living and dieing, simultaneously, throughout a lifetime. When the two phases of the processes of life are balanced there is an imperative state of satisfactory health in the living object, whether animal or plant.

Forces of nature

The great forces of nature are so impressively expressed in

the times of the year when each of the phases of constructive and destructive processes are dominant. It can only be guessed as to just which, if not all, of the forms of energy are responsible for the great surge of power for growth when spring and summer come, and for their recession as the lower temperatures of autumn and winter arrive. Rain, snow, ice, moisture (in all states), formation of solids, liquids, gases, all tangible and intangible energies of all sorts, and every arrangement of matter with resulting manifestations are the result of some state of matter in the universal cycle.

It is unfortunate that most of man's attempts to artificially utilize energy is for destructive purposes. He seems to not be interested in research designed to discover the secrets of constructive energies, - all of which seem productive of life.

Effects of fear

Fear excites a very definite and considerable minimum of muscular tension which is increased with the increase of the fear. The resulting muscular contraction approximates the two vertebrae forming each of the twenty-four joints of the vertebral column formed by them and has a similar effect upon the first cervical vertebra and the occipital bone forming a part of the base of the skull. The undesirable effect of approximating these bones is mechanical pressure on nerve trunks, two of which (one on each side) lie between the bones of each joint of the spine. This pressure on the nerve trunks, reducing the capacity for transmitting nerve impulses over the nerve and its branches, thus depriving the functional cells of the area in which nerve trunk and its branches are distributed and over which the nerve stimulated and function, --according to their particular classification.

Energy influence

All functioning ordinarily begins with the sensory nerve-cell being stimulated from environmental unneutrality and may involve only two or three (or a great many) nerve cells constituting the neural arc which leads to a nerve center and out again to muscle or gland cells in which all neural arcs terminate. This is where movement of some kind is induced to do the work required to restore energy (necessary to stimulate cells and coordinate their functioning) is transmitted.

Every manifestation (desirable or undesirable) of change, fixity, density, arrangement, color, volume, chemical composition or temperature (and every quality of matter) is the result of energy influence.

The constructive and destructive phases of energy may be, for general consideration, equal, - either offsetting the other so that there is a balance in nature's forces. However, like the atmosphere that surrounds the earth (which is more or less uniform), there are fluctuations (from time to time) at different places. For life to manifest in matter, there must be at least an approximate equality of the two energy phases (constructive and destructive). And for living processes to continue, there cannot be too wide deviations from equality of the two phases of energy. For growth, the environment must be conditioned to meet the demands of the constructive phase of the processes essential to life.

In a satisfactory state of health, anabolism (constructive) and catabolism (destructive) would be approximately equal in each 24 hour period. In a satisfactory environment these phases of metabolism would be approximately equal in each 24 hour period. Should anabolism (cellular ingestion) exceed catabolism (cellular elimination), the ingested substance would be assimilated and held in the cell as fat or other cellular protoplasm, or in a refined state as potential energy, to be released upon the application of a stimulus to the cell.

Any unneutrality in the environment (whether mechanical, chemical or thermal) will stimulate the sensory nerve cells of the area. They, in turn, will project nerve impulses to other functional cells which will become neutral in the original area where the environmental unneutrality initiated the functional cycle.

It is through this process that life exists and changes are made.

139

Chapter XII

THE CHIROPRACTIC SPINE

There is the spine, --then there is the "chiropractic spine."

A unique approach

In this chapter on the chiropractic spine, why do we differentiate and insist that the chiropractic view of the spine is different? It is not the acknowledged and supported description of the anatomy of the spine with which chiropractic science takes issue. It is the interrelated circumstance of function that opens up conjecture as to a variance from previously accepted conclusions.

Since it is the chiropractic profession that has made the public spine conscious, then it is for the chiropractic profession to continue to be aware and continue to develop those aspects related to the spine that have been studied by chiropractic science and add to this study the profound information that never before took shape in this advanced direction until chiropractic studies introduced this as a major field of learning in connection with health.

This chapter will concern itself not with just the commonly accepted basics of the spine but with those areas where chiropractic has exposed the importance of the spine in health matters of a general nature that relate both directly and indirectly to the spine.

Spine/nerve interference

The study of the spine is naturally caught up in the study of the nerve system which is an integral part of spine functioning. And it is the nerve system, of course, that is responsible for the coordination of body functions related to sickness and to health. The actual focal point of concern, then, for the chiropractic physician, is the nerve system.

The major emphasis of chiropractic science is upon the neurological influence upon total body health. And it is this whole body concern of the chiropractor that qualifies him/her as a chiropractic physician, entering into procedures to accomplish neurological corrections that will favorably influence the health of the patient.

Articulation deviations

In reviewing the spine and its neurological components, it can be seen, basically, that there are normal ranges of movement within the spine that the chiropractic physician must consider. There are also normal static positions at which the articulation is found at rest. And when these two factors are deviated to any degree there will be the element of 'subluxation' that, correspondingly, comes into effect.

Chiropractic contributions

In consideration of the spine and its grave importance, it has been the chiropractic profession that has been responsible for the development of palpation into an exacting procedure that employs the tacticle senses in such manner as to elicit information concerning the positioning and motion of the vertebral articulations for example. In fact, a specialized procedure in this connection with which all chiropractic doctors are familiar is the concentrated attention upon this area by Henri Gillet, DC, of Brussels, Belgium, particularly. Dr Gillet has, in connection with his studies, also directed attention to 'spinal fixations.'

In connection with the developments related to fixation-consciousness in the chiropractic profession, Dr Clarence W Weiant, some twenty years ago, commented: "An outgrowth of the work of the Belgians has been to discover something we suspected for a long time. The conclusion: That anything you do to any point in the spine changes conditions at other points in the spine, and they report instances in which an atlas adjustment releases a sacroiliac and in which an adjustment of the sacroiliac releases an atlas fixation. It works both ways, but not always, and that is why it is important to check by a fixat-

tion test -because when it doesn't happen that way-- then you
need to give an additional adjustment."

Palpation

Palpation can be conducted in standing, seated or lying positions and is a major area of study in all chiropractic academic
institutions.

Palpation can play an important role, also, in aiding determination of what areas will be radiologically viewed.

Curvatures

In addition to the localized articulation disturbance, the chiropractor is also called upon to be very knowledgeable concerning both normal and deviated curvatures and the way they
relate to a need for corrective procedure.

Therapy considerations

While the medical concept related to the spine --and even to
neurological problems-- has been one of concern, primarily, for
the area of pain, chiropractic has, naturally, in its overall concept, merely considered the pain-factor as a part of the whole
picture and not the major item of concern.

Research

The research work of C H Suh, PhD, at the University of
Colorado, Boulder City, Colorado, is helping to establish the
chiropractic concept of the importance of full attention to the
spine and neurological connections in health matters. Most references have been under the heading of 'Biomechanics of the
spine.'

Research conclusions have been very rewarding and contributory toward better understanding of chiropractic concepts when the scientific community is made aware of these
ongoing developments.

142

Spinal hygiene

The chiropractic profession, in its concern for the spine, has not only been engaged in developing means by which correction can be made to allow recovery in health problems but must be recognized for the additional information being developed that aids in the prevention of ill health through a respect for spinal hygiene.

With chiropractic awareness of the vertebral column as a somewhat delicate (in the sense of sensitivity) yet perfectly constructed and physiologically dependable in its mechanical functioning, and having the specific function of supporting and protecting the spinal cord and projecting nerves (most extremely important), the chiropractic physician becomes obligated to create public knowledge in this matter so that there will be a public awareness of the importance of proper spinal hygiene as well as the need for attention to the spine when not functionally satisfactory.

The subluxation

Responding to a need for focussing more attention upon the chiropractic concentration upon the vertebral subluxation, as per the advice of J F McAndrews, DC, president of Palmer Chiropractic College, the WORLD-WIDE REPORT editor, Paul Smallie, DC, authored and published in the November, 1983 issue, the following:

It wasn't so long ago that a concerned focus of attention in the area of subluxations developed with the entrance of chiropractic representation in governmental recognition for Medicare purposes.

Although the interest at that time was more in the nature of the profession being compelled to elaborate a bit on what constituted subluxation, so that the legislators would have, at least, a basic idea of what is involved, it was surprising, at the time, that description of just what constituted a subluxation

143

was not just a simple definition with which all were familiar and all were agreed. There was brain-drain involved with putting together something that would be acceptable to everyone and still be able to describe for those unfamiliar with the term subluxation, just what was meant. So what the chiropractic officials came up with was this:

A subluxation is the alteration of the normal dynamics, anatomical or physiological relationships of contiguous structures.

They described the extensiveness of its manifestations in this way.

In evaluation of this complex phenomenon, we find that it has or may have biomechanical pathophysiological, clinical, radiologic, and other manifestations.

As to the reason for concern with this 'phenomenon,' it was stated that subluxations are of clinical significance as they are affected by or evoke abnormal physiological responses in neuromusculoskeletal structures and/or other body systems.

In considering the possible radiological manifestations of subluxations, it was stated that it is important to emphasize that clinical judgement is necessary to determine the necessity of exposing a patient to the potential hazards of ionizing radiation.

It was added that the importance of exposures, beside the evaluation of subluxations, was the determination of the evidence of other pathologies.

It was also added that the radiographic procedures necessary to determine possible fractures, malignancies, etc., may not be the specific view needed to evaluate the possible radiological manifestations of subluxation. And it was also advised at the time that when subluxation can be evaluated by other means, it may be prudent to avoid radiation exposure.

As is known, however, Medicare still insisted on the 'as shown

144

by x-ray' clause and so it continues to be enforceable as THE diagnostic factor that establishes subluxations as existing.

Classifying

In classifying subluxations, these radiological manifestations were noted:

Static Intersegmental subluxations: Flexion, malposition, Extension malposition, Lateral flexion malposition, Rotational malposition, Anterolisthesis, Re trolisthesis, Lateralisthesis, Altered interosseous spacing, Osseous foraminal encroachment. Kinetic intersegmental subluxation, Hypomobility.

Kinetic intersegmental subluxation: Hypomobility (fixation subluxation), Hypermobility, Aberrant motion.

Sectional subluxations: Scoliosis and/or curves secondary to musculature imbalance. Scoliosis and/or alteration of curves secondary to musculature imbalance. Scoliosis and/or alteration of curves secondary or structural asymmetries, Decompensation of adaptational curvatures, Abnormalities of motion.

X-ray and the subluxation

Writing on the subject in 1972, Dr Frank A Hoffman, of the National Chiropractic College faculty, observed that there has been in addition to the vast writing on the subject many descriptive definitions that caused much confusion in the scientific world.

Standards to confirm a subluxation diagnosis were set up by an ACA Review Commission, at the time, declaring the subluxation to be, roughly, an incomplete or partial dislocation.

It was also concluded that a spinal subluxation can be defined as hypermobility or hypomobility of one or more motor units producing a physiological reaction.

It was emphasized that in using the subluxation term, there

145

should be neurological and neurophysiological correlation noted.

Enumeration of evidences of spinal subluxations diagnosed by x-ray were listed as:

Alteration of Georges' line, Alteration of Hedley's line, Facet gapping, Aberrant motion, McNab's line. Disc wedging with disrelationship, Foraminal encroachment, Intervertebral subluxations that are further divided into the following two classifications:

Static Flexion, Extension, Lateral, Rotary, Spondylolisthesis, Retrolisthesis, Lateralisthesis, Altered interosseous spacing, Kinetic Hypermobility, Hypomobility.

Subluxation research

Heading the ACA Department of Research in the late 60s, Dr Henry Higley came up with some very vital conclusions for the profession that served to place the profession on a more accepted scientific basis in the matter of substantiating the existence of subluxations.

Here are excerpts from some of the conclusions of the pioneering DC spinal subluxation researcher, Dr Higley.

Investigators within and outside the chiropractic profession seemed in agreement in corroborating the following conclusions.

As a result of trauma or muscular force, misalignment and fixation of the segments of the spine (subluxations), may result in inflammatory processes with possible edema and compression of the nerves emerging from the intervertebral foramina.

When the inflammatory process reaches a certain degree of severity and continues for several weeks, the compression of the nerve trunk leads to degeneration of the nerve fibers. The nerve distal to the constriction becomes smaller in diameter,

146

changes in shape, and carries fewer nerve fibers to innervate the parts supplied by such a nerve. Muscles subjected to this reduced nerve supply lose some of their efficiency.

As far back as 1968, Dr Higley was calling for the profession to organize and publicize for the benefit of the world a knowledge of what the detection and correction of nerve compression means. But there was never a great response to this plea until more recently when Drs Flesia and Riekman have come up with the encouragement to make everyone, everywhere, very conscious of the importance of detecting and correcting the vertebral subluxation.

The plea has been for massive support for such declarations by the profession.

Dr Higley, alerting the profession to the need to stress greater attention upon the knowledge they had gained in connection with the subluxation observed, "Perhaps the most important thing that we are learning is the presence of prolonged nerve pressure is a much more serious problem than is generally considered."

Dr Higley's plea was that they make the world aware that just as soon as the presence of nerve pressure is detected, there should be steps taken to relieve such pressure just as soon as possible to prevent further damage.

The Henry Higley name should never be forgotten among the greats who worked arduously and intellectually to accomplish what was needed to help place the profession on a more scientific basis.

Dedicated men like Dr Higley dug into the intricacies of the subluxation and made the knowledge available only to have it denied the importance it warranted.

In reviewing the conclusions of those like Dr Henry Higley, the profession would be wise to also reintroduce for itself the conclusions from the very sound and supportable research of

Dr Earl Homewood in his masterful presentation of the "Neurodynamics of the Vertebral Subluxation" that elaborated on the neurology, the physiology and the mechanics of the subluxation.

The writing of Dr W D Harper should also not be overlooked in any search for evidence for DCs to support the need for intense concentration upon the subluxation.

It was Dr Harper who tended to elaborate upon and pin down some of the studious observations made by D D Palmer to help to popularize such conclusions and direct the attention of the profession to their importance.

It was Dr Harper who said of D D Palmer that it was he who established a common factor in all disease processes and advised the profession that the greatest monument that we could leave to the founder of this profession would be to establish his principles as the reason for this remarkable performance.
(This was the end of the WORLD-WIDE REPORT article)

Subluxation and D D Palmer

In arriving at a working concept as to what constitutes a subluxation, it was T F Ratledge who volunteered this concept:

"The word 'subluxation' in order to have a specific chiropractic meaning-- must be in support of the discovery by D D Palmer, i. e., that obstructive pressure on a nerve or nerves is caused by a vertebral subluxation only when the relation of the positions of contiguous vertebrae are not automatically corrected by complete muscular relaxation following a return of environmental neutrality after cessation of the stimulatory stress; chemical, mechanical or thermal.

"All chiropractic definitions should, at least, imply the purpose of correcting vertebral subluxations.

"All subluxations are primarily protective, if temporary. Otherwise, they exert some degree of obstruction to transmission of nerve energy and proportionately impair function of the tissues to which the impinged nerve or nerves may supply, normally, stimulatory energy impulses. Protoplasmic adaptation is the process by which subluxations become more or less fixed unless expansion of the intervertebral cartilages automatically correct this when muscular contractions stop, either from exhaustion or because of environmental neutralization. The elasticity of intervertebral cartilages automatically reestablishes normal relations between approximated vertebrae in proportion to decreased muscular contraction, thus, correcting nerve pressures."

Terminology

Ronald J Watkins, DC, writing in the Canadian Chiropractic Association Journal, in 1968, covered "Subluxation Terminology Since 1746," and reported:

"Hieronymus in 1746 wrote 'Subluxation of joints is recognized by lessened motion of joints, by slight change in the position of the articulating bones and by pain...most displacements of vertebrae are subluxations rather than luxations."

After this introduction, Dr Watkins followed by quoting the consensus of dictionary opinion, "disrelationship between two adjacent articulatory bones in which the articulating surfaces have not lost contact."

Dr Watkins further introduces his subject in stating, "D D Palmer insisted that the word subluxation be applied to the intervertebral disrelationship amounting to less than a locked dislocation but he maintained at the same time that there is a functional response within the nervous system resulting from this structural disrelationship..."

Dr Watkins does much to clarify some of the misimpressions of the past when he describes the common understanding of the classic subluxation, chiropracticly considered, to be "a tilt rotation or both between two adjacent vertebrae," and adds "Contrary to some definitions in the past, the subluxation is of a joint, not of a bone; hence it is not necessary to have disrelationship both above and below a vertebra to call the condition a subluxation." And this is important in considering vertebral subluxations because of the tendency of some to attempt to discredit subluxation existence.

Dr Watkins enumerates a large number of variations in degrees and relationships that would constitute a subluxation and includes "abnormal patterns of movement" as "quite definitely subluxations" in the dictionary sense of the term.

Dr Watkins suggests clarifying by use of standardized definitions broken down into the following subdivisions:

SUBLUXATION - Static or kinetic (less than luxation) disrelationship between two adjacent articulating joint surfaces." The following types have been observed: A) Tilt with disc wedging; rotation with disc torque or both together; B) Limitation of some motions with free excursion of others (partial fixation), C) Loss of all motions (total fixation); D) Normal neutral position but reversed motion in some directions (paradoxical - usually a sympton); E) Normal neutral and extreme positions but subject to erratic, jumpy motion during shifts of positions (usually a symptom).

*Observe, says Dr Watkins, that these descriptions mention nothing of occlusion, interference or neurological implications. This avoids differentiations of 'subluxations' from 'distortion' which is impossible on x-ray films.

NEUROPATHY - Any neurological dysfunction; including earlier dysfunction than the histologically demonstrable 'dystrophy.' The term neuropathy is now used by scientists generally to imply slowing of the speed of impulse transmission plus altered reflexes and paresthesias. It is found consistently in diabetes mellitus, rheumatoid arthritis and increasing, as technology is refined, in all the degenerative pathologies.

Hence the classic chiropractic definition of a subluxation can be better stated as an 'intervertebral subluxation with consequent neuropathy.' Since this is definitely not always the case, there are the following combinations seen and described:

1) Subluxation with minor muscle imbalance with no consequent neuropathy. (These usually clear quickly and easily - no vasodilation failure); 2) Subluxation with consequent neuropathy. (Classic chiropractic specialty); 3) Subluxation as a symptom of a neuropathy. (Local or remote) This type subluxation as a symptom can initiate further neuropathies to become a complex chain).

Any neuropathy can also exist as a self perpetuating vicious circle, after the original subluxation has physically disappeared. This emphatically illustrates the critical importance of the time factor. Each patient is the sum total of all prior neurological experience.

The listings of subluxations with their brief description (rotation, lateral tilting and flexion or extension) should be made on any x-ray study. Their clinical significance and reason for adjusting must be made by muscle and motion palpation, test pressures, trial adjustments and evaluation of various neurological responses.

The observations of Dr Watkins, herein concluded, bring one closer to the intricacies involved in the ongoing exploring and refinement of knowledge of subluxations.

In helping to determine how extensively one might evaluate the existence, influence and effects of subluxation, Dr T L Shrader produced the following questionnaire that tends to sum up just what it is the chiropractic physician is interested in under the heading of concern for the subluxation:

1. Would you describe the particular subluxation we are concerned with in this study, and indicate the manner in which the various structures have changed from normal in their relationship or function. (X-ray, drawings, anatomical models)
2. What subjective complaint do patients usually experience

151

with this condition.

3. What history would be typical of the circumstances and mode of onset for this condition.

4. Would you describe or demonstrate examining procedures used to establish the diagnosis of this particular subluxation.

A) Physical examination
  1. Visual observation, palpation, motion testing
  2. Neurological
  3. Orthopedic
  4. Muscle testing and therapy localization
  5. Instrument
B) Laboratory testing
C) X-ray
D) Other

5. In addition to the possibility that a subluxation may be part of an abnormal reflex syndrome, there are other complications or even contra-indicating conditions of circumstances which affect a doctor's decisions as the use of adjustive technic. Among such examples as congenital anomalies, degenerative, inflammatory and pathological states, and traumas, are any especially common or peculiar to the structures involved in this study.

6. Would you describe any visceral problems which may be associated with this subluxation.

7. Describe the specific objectives of your technic maneuvers, and how they relate to the subluxation.

A) What changes in structural relationships do you intend to make with your adjustive maneuver.

B) If fixation is involved, what muscle or tissue is the offender.

C) In what way can changes in discs, cartilages, ligaments, and bursae contribute to the existence of this subluxation.

8. With any of the above conditions and therapeutic objectives in mind, would you describe your technic selection and its application.
INCLUDE:
  A Unique equipment required
  B Patient and doctor position relative to both testing and

152

adjusting.

C Preparatory maneuvers or provision for traction,counter-force, resistance, or relaxation.

D The adjustive maneuvers - contacts, line of drive, timing and force estimate.

E Post-adjustment testing for successful application.

F Necessary adjunctive procedures, care and advice.

9. Under circumstances in which the usual technic may not be indicated, what are the alternatives.

10. Under what conditions is the prognosis favorable.

11. Under what conditions is the prognosis unfavorable.

12. What sources and references have you relied upon in providing information for this study.

-end of

(ACA TECHNIC COUNCIL QUESTIONNAIRE)

In late 1966, with the assistance of Daniel W Carlson, DC, Henry G Higley, DC, director of the Department of Research of Los Angeles Chiropractic College and Director of the Department of Research and Statistics of the American Chiropractic Association, published an article under the heading of "Physiology of a Subluxation." It described as the purpose of the article a reexamining of the physiological aspects of a subluxation in the light of increasing experimental, clinical, and surgical evidence attesting to the existence of such a physiological phenomena as the subluxation.

The research article looked at impingement, irritation and altered blood supply and tended to show more weight of conclusive evidence in the area of irritation and altered blood supply. The area of impingement, while supporting the "classical chiropractic approach to the problem" found it necessary to divide conclusions into several sub-classifications and interpretations by different researchers.

Briefly stated, said the article, "impingement includes pressure from internal or external sources, compression, and fibrous encroachment."

153

Functional concept

Ten years ago, David C Drum, DC, published a "Functional Concept of Vertebral Subluxations." He wrote:

"A spinal subluxation is any disruption of the normal mechanics of the functional unit of the spine."

Dr Drum described fixation subluxations that are reducible by chiropractic adjustment as being, "by far, the most common motor unit abnormality."

The important message of Dr Drum's reserach was to the effect that in the fixation-type subluxation, "nothing is out of place." Segments, he explains, in fact, are more accurately described as being too much "in place," their full expression of movement being blocked. And he adds, "The nature of this spinal subluxation lends it to virtually all forms of manipulative techniques because the therapeutic goal is simply mobilization."

In 1974, William D Shephard, DC, of Oshkosh, Wisconsin, regarded the area of compensation or strain as it relates to the subluxation and volunteered the observation, "We must admit that the majority of people are not adjusted promptly after subluxation and their bodies must compensate..."

Dr Shephard describes compensation as "anything the body does to decrease the irritation of a nerve in a subluxation." He suggests that compensation takes place immediately and is consistent, allowing a study through such consistence.

Dr Shephard describes the tendency of the spine to coil into a spiral. This introduces the element of third dimensional analysis often neglected in the overall characterization of the extent of changes in the spine under subluxation conditions.

Dr Shephard says "Most of us see patients at a point where the compensation has been strained in some fashion. This strain loosens the compensatory locks and allows tilted and

distorted joints to move in odd unnatural movements which ir
ritate the nerve root at the strain site and cause pain."

What Dr Shephard is suggesting is that in adjustive procedures, the chiropractor is first concerned with the compensatory circumstances that have been created and then being in
position, as a follow-up, to be concerned with the subluxation
as it existed before compensation entered the picture.

Dr Shephard refers to the muscluar weaknesses involved in
subluxations and offers the conclusion that such weaknesses
observed "will not clear till both compensation and subluxation are cleared."

Chapter XIII

CHIROPRACTIC ADJUSTING

<u>Adjust</u>, v. The act of bringing into more proper relationship the vertebrae in the spinal column. The purpose is to eliminate the unsatisfactory degree of obstructive pressure upon nerves that lie in the intervertebral foramina. These are the foraminal obstructions that are formed by approximation of the intervertebral notches. These foramina are subject to very considerable fluctuation in size during flexion of the spine. And when there is general muscular tension, --in which instance there is general compression of the intervertebral cartilages-- it is then that obstructive pressure is exerted upon the nerves which lie in the foramina.

<u>Adjustment</u>, n. A state of being in which there is no obstructive pressure on nerves.

<u>Adjusting</u>, v. A process by which the state of adjustment is attained.It occurs from forcing vertebral change. One instance is that of permitting the intervertebral cartilages to expand. These cartilages are elastic and automatically expand unless they are compressed by too long sustained compression. The adjusting changes the relationship in the vertebral articulation and, thereby, increases the size of the openings in which the nerves lie. Correspondingly, this reduces existing obstructive nerve pressure, permitting uninhibited transmission of nerve energy. And this is the purpose of the adjusting.

Importance

Adjusting the spine is incorporated into chiropractic as its most integral part. It is inseparable from the whole science of chiropractic. Therefore, it is incorrect when lecturers and writers give adjusting a minor role relative to its place in chiropractic or refer to it as a "therapy of chiropractic."

Adjusting is the "IT" of the art of chiropractic science.

Purpose

T F Ratledge simplified what was basically the underlying factor as to why adjusting was the major indicated procedure. He said that the primary purpose of all effort to apply the chiropractic principle is to remove obstructive pressure from nerves. And this is done so that up to 100% of nerve energy may be delivered to such areas as needed for optimumu function in the body.

Functional activity has been described as the only way that the needs for environmental neutralization can be acquired. And it seems there is no other need for functioning as far as keeping the body alive and healthy. So functional adequacy seems to be the answer to sustaining health. This is the functional activity that is called into play to meet all fluctuations in environment changes.

Obstruction removal

As to better measures to accomplish the reestablishing of adequate functional activity , it is obvious that if obstructive interference has been the causative factor, then removal should be the remedy.

Procedure

Without question, it is best to proceed as specifically as possible. And pressure directed to the involved vertebrae would be the most logical and has proved the most effective.

More technically, the entire articulation is more relative than just the vertebral structure, itself. It is the functional unity with which the chiropractor is concerned, rather than just the bony structure, itself.

The spine as a spring

In the early days of pioneering in the development of adjustive procedures related to the spine, a simplified but profound example was used in aiding an adjustor to experience a tangible comparison to convey a clearly portrayed concept.

Dr Herb E Weiser, then Dean of the Texas Chiropractic College found that directing adjustive force to a spine could be improved while thinking of it as a form of spring. He said, at the time in this early date of establishing adjusting concepts, "When we adjust this column, we should keep in mind that we are adjusting a spring. If we approach the art of adjusting the spinal column from the angle of adjusting the leaves of a spring it will lead us into a wide field of new technique and methods of making analysis. And he further elaborated, "In the normal weight bearing positions, most of the strain is on the bodies of the vertebrae, the articulating processes acting merely as stabilizers. When, however, the curves become abnormally exaggerated, an excessive amount of weight is thrown upon the articular processes in the cervical and lumbar regions, while in the thoracic region the bodies become more compressed, anteriorly."

Early-day tables

Another early-day concept in adjusting that drifted out of vogue –yet had much going for it as an adjusting aid– came out of the Texas College, also. It was in the form of an adjusting table built for Dr James Drain, college president. It was conceived in the form of an elevated convex shape, superiorly. It allowed the patient to lie upon it with a tendency toward more openness of the spinal articulations. The back became more relaxed and arched upward to open up the articulations, further, before applying adjusting pressure.

Among the tables for adjusting of that period that have dropped out of common usage –though still retaining their basic advantages-- was the Ratledge-conceived,Carver-modified table that was further improved upon by Dr Frank Mussler. It allowed a release of the support from the pelvic area on down by placing this area on a hinge that allowed downward moverment for low back adjusting. Newer models neglected to include this important movement area.

In analyzing the adjustic effort and physics involved in the adjusting procedures as presented under Ratledge College direction, it was clear that there is a maximum distribution of pressure exerted upon the surface of the body and tissues between the surface and the spinous process of the vertebra to be moved and, of course, the minimum of mechanical stimulation in applying the procedure.

This is conceived to guard against irritating tissues in applying force.

With the above described contact, with relaxed wrist and shoulder joints, but with fixed elbow, with the arm straight, the adjustor, with a little experience, will detect any movement between the vertebra contacted and the one above (or in the case of the atlas, will detect any movement between atlas and occiput) and being perfectly coordinated in the muscles used, may (at will) relax, instantly, and there will be no danger of applying force to any degree beyond that necessary to move the vertebra.

Such procedure would obviate all possibility of moving a vertebra too far, irrespective of how much effort was put into the process up to that point.

The skilled adjustor, by neuro-muscular coordination, senses vertebral movement, relaxes elbow, changes the thrust, or stiff arm stress, to a spring action from which no unnecessary continuation of force is involved.

In making an atlas adjustment with the above adjustment, with the above described contact, there is --in the beginning of the effort- an upward (superior) direction of the pressure, but with the wrist and shoulder joints relaxed and freely moveable. This changes as the body of the adjustor swings parallel with the spine toward the head and continues to so-change until the atlas movement is sensed and the elbow joint relaxed.

The upward movement of the head takes up any slack that may be in the capsules and ligaments of the occipito-atlantal joint and makes any movement of the atlas instantly perceptible.

The swinging movement of the body, from below, upward, from a point considerably too low, has another great advantage, in that as pressure is applied from the beginning, brings

159

the pressure to the proper angle, somewhere in the arc.

It is impossible for the patient to guess the direction of the thrust and to offer direct muscular resistance. In this way, the distress of muscular resistance by the patient is minimized.

As most of the patient distress is due to his own involuntary resistance to the physical stress of making an adjustment of vertebral joints.

The lower of the two vertebrae exerting obstructive pressure on a nerve, because of articular surface directions, is the proper point of stress in making any correction of such nerve pressure.

The palm contact, directly upon the lower vertebrae in all subluxations is the most practical and involved the very minimum of chance of injury.

It is desirable to proceed as specifically as possible in the correction of obstructive nerve pressure. Pressure directed to one vertebra at a time, and to the lower of the two between which such pressure exists, is the most logical and most effective procedure for intentional correction.

No attempt to correct nerve pressure should be made until after thorough examination, noting general and local variation from normal relations of spinal area, and after palpation of the entire spine to determine the individual relation of the two vertebrae forming any joint in the patient's condition. Thus, conclusions, not diagnoses, are reached and problems of correction considered.

The palm contact · directly upon the body surface--, with the fifth metacarpal directly upon the spinal nerves is preferable to other contacts for correction in any part of the vertebral column.

Grostic

The Grostic Procedure had its origins in the Palmer Specific Upper Cervical technique. It was one of several techniques that developed as a result of efforts to standardize chiropractic procedures and methods. Much of this effort to standardize the profession was the result of a group of chiropractors under the direction of BJ Palmer. The group, known as the Palmer Standardized Chiropractic Council founded by Roy G Labachotte, DC, of Redwood City, California, provided a forum at which research and new ideas could be presented and exchanged.

Dr John F Grostic was one of the members of this organization. He, along with other chiropractors, would present research and ideas at Council meetings. Meetings evolved into Palmer's Pre-Lyceum program. This was the initial phase of Grostic procedures.

Grostic Procedure is primarily a measurement system. The x-ray analysis is the core of the procedure and has remained as a constant for over 30 years. Adjusting methods, however, have changed. The Palmer Toggle became a modified shorter and lighter thrust. Travelling point is less than ¼-inch during the thrust.

There is continued evaluation, and new adjustive methods are continuously being tested.

Sacro-Occipital Technic

Well known within the chiropractic profession along with other technics such as Gonstead and any number of others is the technic of Major B De Jarnette, DC, called Sacro-Occipital.

Simply stated, says Dr De Jarnette, Sacro-Occipital Technic is a method of chiropractic that seeks the adjustment that will do the patient the most good in the least period of time and remain effective the longest time possible. It seeks to remove the excessive stimuli as quickly as possible. It seeks to give that adjustment which will produce the least discomfort and the greatest sense of well being.

Says Dr De Jarnette, further, "The chiropractic subluxation is not a slipped vertebra which has placed pressure upon a nerve. In an adjustment, says Dr De Jarnette, further, much more takes place than the concussion of forces.

Dr De Jarnette describes the subluxation as "something very much alive. It can be compared to a microorganism that is living upon tissues other than its own. The subluxation has vitality and it takes this vitality from the tissues which oppose its presence. The subluxation has 'motion,' and it derives this motion from the component parts which try to stabilize it.

The chiropractic subluxation is not a vertebra that is slipped,

161

pressed, shoved, forced, driven, catapulted or otherwise mis-
placed or displaced with its neighbor above or below and is not
a fixed thing which responds not, but lies quietly and presses
upon delicate tissues.

Dr De Jarnette explains correction with the word motion and
says " Nothing else you can say so well explains what you do
when you give a chiropractic adjustment to the vertebra
by its motion creates stimuli which, in turn, creates pain and
disease. Your adjustment, if properly given, controls motion
and removes stimuli resulting from motion. Motion is the primary product of a vertebral subluxation for only motion can
create inflammation through irritation. And irritation causes

Dr De Jarnette has said of adjusting, "Thousands of chiropractors are trying to learn new adjustments when in reality
they need to learn where and when to use the adjustments
they now know and use so skillfully."

Mortimer Levine

Adding to the above thought are the words of Mortimer Levine, DC, who was chairman of the Department of Chiropractic of the Chiropractic Institute of New York and author of
the text, The Structural Approach To Chiropractic. He said:
"It is unrealistic to think that we can directly negotiate the
function of the nervous system with an adjustment. The business of the nervous system is the nervous system's business!
The chiropractor's concern is with the restoration and maintenance of structural integrity. The doctor is unable to regulate function except as it is done indirectly by adjusting a
faulty structural condition and by advising the patient to adjust his way of life so as to avoid and minimize distorting influences."

Dr Levine further added, "Chiropractic's rationale is hardly
based on the fact that its adjustive techniques are applied with
a sudden force. It is the reason why these techniques are applied that distinguishes chiropractic from other healing disciplines. We are not able to place parts of the body into their exact relationships. But we are able to release the holding elements which are preventing the parts from assuming their normal juxtapositions."

"The correction of distortion and restoration of normal anatomical relationships," declared Dr Levine, "are dependent not only on what we do to the body, but on how the body responds to what we have done. Articulations are dynamic mechanisms. Their function is movement. Hence, the static view of a pair of interlocking articulations at any particular instant is virtually meaningless as is the degree of rotation of a single vertebra at a given instant. The moment the patient steps away from the position he assumed for the radiographer's convenience, the vertebra in question will have assumed a new relative position (unless the vertebra is in fixation)."

Dr Levine concluded, "As a working principle, the primary concern in giving an adjustment is not to establish position but to reestablish movement."

Janse description

In a series of articles on vertebral subluxations and adjustment several years ago, Dr Joseph J Janse now president emeritus of National Chiropractic College, presented a description of the vertebral subluxation followed by what is accomplished in the chiropractic adjustment.

"A vertebral subluxation may be interpreted as an off-centering of a vertebral segment, in relation to the one above and below and usually at the extreme or slightly beyond the normal range of movement. As a result the vertebra is no longer capable of the physiological demands of normal movement, resulting in a variable degree of fixation, vertebral joint strain, a pathological altering of the diameters of the intervertebral foraminae, with possible consequent nerve trunk impingement, paraforaminal congestions and eventual development of adhesions.

"The chiropractic adjustment helps to remove nerve impingement at the intervertebral foramen; helps to relieve the tension and traction upon the spinal nerve trunk attending an undue widening of the intervertebral foramen as produced by subluxation; represents the most effective way of 'breaking' the fixation characteristic of all types of vertebral and pelvic sub-

163

luxations, the most effective means of affecting structural correction of the human biped spine; serves most effectively in maintaining the postural and myotonic proficiency of the human as a biped, serves in maintaining the myotatic reflexes and variances so essential to effective postural integrity and good health, the most concise means of physiologically stimulating the venous drainage, an element so very important in dissipating inimical toxic accumulations, especially within the central gray substance; the most effective way of restoring the structural relationship of the vertebral and pelvic segments; the most effective way of lending to the nervous system a manner of physiological stimulation that tends to normalize all body functions."

Extensive technique awareness

All the above references to adjusting variations from different chiropractic authorities is not intended to imply that there is some pointed reason for inclusion of these, alone. This, of course –as is known–, is not in the area of full information within the vast storehouse area of adjusting information for the profession. Far from it!

The intent, here, has been only in the sense of familiarizing the reader with just a few of the many, many chiropractic approaches that have, naturally, developed over the years.

Adjusting tables

Although chiropractic adjusting tables have become fairly well standardized with the predominant models like Zenith and the newer modified McManus and others becoming more popular it is good to listen to some of the table recommendations of chiropractic educators like T F Ratledge who enjoyed long experience with dedicated study and with experience developing tables that had specific functional purposes. Dr Ratledge believed all sections should be independently flexible and hinged accordingly. with freedom for fixity or rigidity. And he encouraged an arrangement in which the front and rear sections would be subject to elevation and to lowering of each.The middle section should allow total lowering, alone or in consonance with the tilting of either or both, front and rear sections. The middle section should be hinged at rear end of the front section. There should be rigid joints, crosswise, at the discretion of the adjustor, at the level of clavicle and manubrium and at front end of rear section, approximately at the level of the hip joints.

"Rigidity at the level of the clavicle and manubrium is a must in adjusting lower cervicals and upper thoracics.

"Both front and back sections released and free to tilt, in unison with the released and lowered middle section, facilitates lumbar adjusting. This position flexes the lower thoracic and lumbar posteriorly, thus offsetting the otherwise constant tendency to forward flexion and stooping posture.

"A too soft upholstering does not permit specific vertebral movement. The springy nature of such prevents specific adjustment just as a springy board makes driving a nail difficult or impossible.

"Certain and proper resistance is necessary to perform specific movement of any particular vertebra.

"A committee investigating the general proposition of vertebral, specific and intentional, adjusting should have as a consultant, an engineer, –to analyze the potential stresses possible with different positions of the patient.

"The subject of chiropractic adjusting tables demands the most thorough research by men qualified by education and experience to understand the objectives of chiropractic adjusting...

Chapter XIV

HEALTH

Health education

A chiropractic education equipts one for general health practice. Such practice is not in the sense of a specialty. There is a "whole person-care" involvement because of the potential associations and coordination of function in all areas of the entire human body which, after all, is a unit. It should not be separated into that which gives an impression that one activity of the human body acts alone and independent of its other parts.

Influences

Sickness is a negative state of the body and implies only functional failure to corresponding degrees of intensity of unneutrality of the environment and resulting degenerative processes.

Functional failure -throughout life- is the one condition that is responsible for all the ups and downs in the state of health. Anything that will have an adverse effect upon the human body will produce unsatisfactory metabolic and functional conditions in that body, --automatically--, producing characteristic manifestations. Should the body not have the ability to correct the difference between itself and its environment, then ill health is the normally anticipated consequence.

The very fact of the quality of one's environment not being right is the automatic cause of stimulus exciting functional reaction tending to correct the condition.

A healthy body is one that has the ability to respond to environmental variations. As long as the response is adequate, the body remains healthy. But when the body fails to, functionally, correct the differences between itself and the environment, then that body will become ill.

166

Maint enance of a satisfactory environment is the duty of the individual. How well it is done will determine how well life can be lived and how long it can be lived. But all of it, of course, is also predicated upon maximum potentialities and heredity that must be taken into consideration as influencing factors.

If there can be an accounting for the incidences of stimuli and conditions under which the body can function in environment maintenance, then this opens up an entry into the secrets of life.

Every disease symptom is a manifestation of the body itself. It is explainable on the basis of simple body functioning.

Factors influencing body health can be enumerated under these headings: Time; Duration of injurious factors in the environment, Stress of pressure (positive or negative); Chemical imbalance.

Loss of chemical equilibrium through concentration (or attenuation) in the body fluids (blood and lymph), secretions and exudations or transudations) to a degree beyond the limits of tolerance (or irritability norms) of the body, or any of its cells.

Innate recuperative powers, or vitality and inherited structural characteristics.

Body manifestations, in reacting to unneutralities, would exactly imitate every alleged disease symptom ever observed in disease.

If medical theory of imitating of other diseases in the body were true, none could imitate the body in all its varying manifestations in the processes of adaptation to the stresses of its environment.

All misfortune of humans in matters of health are individual and accidental. The misfortunes are due to what individuals, consciously, do, or fail to do, in the process of adaptation to the environment. An early discovery of this fact would have led to an entirely different approach to health problems.

Being attuned to some natural law permitting living without medicine- under primitive living conditions, it is logical to assume those same laws would be ample under the improved conditions of civilization.

Individuals are healthy because the human body is equipped with the various mechanisms of sense perception necessary to acquiring chemicals for their every need from air, food and water, accurately testing the temperature and mechanical stresses of the environment in order to react in proper function to make adaptations to an ever-changing environment.

Where individuals have been considered hopelessly ill, not responding to the magic of medicine, they have changed their living habits on their own power, making complete recovery. The self-sufficiency of the body in this regard is well illustrated.

Recovery from what is referred to as a cold is, in fact, restoration of satisfactory functional manifestations of the body.

Degrees of temperature

In temperature variations away from the approximate 98.6, if every variation of functional manifestation is to be named, then it would be more accurate to refer to "more" or "less" of every disease. There would be more pneunomia, more typhoid, that would be "caught" by the individual.

Fever

Fever, commonly believed to be some strange form of heat, is just ordinary heat produced by the body at all times. It is not a disease. It is just one of the imperative manifestations (symptoms) of a human body failing - to a particular degree– to function enough to make heat radiation possible as fast as the heat is generated, internally. Fever is a name originated in superstition. It is definitely misleading as descriptive of a mere rise of body temperature.

When the body functions, it incidentally generates heat. When function lessens, there is a corresponding lessening of heat production. These extremes of activity and inactivity produce maximum and minimum of heat in the body. But when functioning is adequate, the body temperature is maintained within one degree change in each 24 hours. It would appear, then, that fever - or even subnormal temperature– is the result of failure of function, -and not of a disease.

Degree is the only difference in fever and in normal temperature.

When dealing with fever, the problem is one of physics. Heat production and dissipation is the problem –and definitely not to induce some wandering chill to attack either the hapless victim of the fever, or attack the fever.

In the matter of fevers, death was hastened upon countless millions through concepts of ignorance. The ministrations were in driving out the evil spirits and use of other similar savage incantations, including the magic of medicine. This was generally accepted as appropriate response. Variations have developed in medical approach, but the prevalent idea of the alleged attackers remains.

Diseases

"Epidemic diseases" have, allegedly, been fought by first identifying the disease. And this was, presumably, in order to know what weapons were to be used against "it." The procedure was, then, to immunize as many people as would, voluntarily, submit to the magic or vaccinations, innoculations, hypodermic shots (introducing fertile disease germs to insure attack by more gentle– germs of the same strain, arousing unsuspecting bodies for which it is necessary to build defenses --or fences-- to keep out the more ferocious diseases –responsible(?) for the epidemic).

The term epidemic is restricted to medical use only and is designated to convey the thought of diseases with power to live, propagate, migrate and attack healthy humans. From the chiropractic point of view, the word is a misnomer as chiropractic science denies the disease entity fable and is not interested in myths.

If the theory of epidemics were correct, then it would be correct to refer to one case of illness as a small epidemic. The more cases would, then, indicate just more of the same.

Each so-called epidemic disease is alleged to attack many people, simultaneously. And it is also alleged that epidemiologists fight and control, exterminating these diseases in certain limited areas. They are thought to be very stubborn, at times ·virulent-, while at other times not as dangerous –even though pandemic as to their seemingly universal existence.

The common cold, malaria, influenza, typhus and typhoid, cholera, - all have been said to fluctuate in the intensity of their attacks. This is a hanover from a pre-science age prevailing before it was known that every manifestation associated with living is due to universal law.

We now know that if one person is injured in a certain way, he will manifest, similarly, as many times as he becomes similarly subjected. If more than one, they too will manifest, similarly. And if there are enough, it becomes an epidemic.

The only difference in the symptoms in any case from another is the intensity of the injurious influence, the energy potential for functional endurance, degree of degenerative change and length of time subjected to injurious agent or condition.

Considering the facts of variable vitality, variable intensities of irritants, or injurious influences, and their duration, it is clear that if any injurious influences should be exerted, simultaneously (upon many individuals), all of them would react similarly and would (under medical therapeutic dispensation), constitute a basis for declaring an epidemic of some disease.

Cause and effect

Factually considered, the logical procedure is to analyze on the basis of cause and effect. As surely as every cause produces an effect, just as surely does every effect become a cause. In other words, there is always a succession of causes and effects.

Given time, chemicals are subject to change, and as long as the body functions it tends to neutralize the chemicals to the standards of individual cellular tolerance. Also, as long as the body functions it tends to maintain the temperature at the average 98.6 and to adjust the fluid pressures within the healthy range of variability. Should factors become sufficiently modified to be outside the ordinary range of variance, it, automatically, becomes an irritant and excites functioning.

Stimulation

Chemicals may stimulate, mildly or violently, or may directly destroy the organized units of the living body. Mild stimulation usually causes the necessary intensity of functional reaction to re-neutralize the chemical, mechanical and thermal irritants affecting the body without undue fatigue. Violent stimulation results in rapid dissipation of the reserve energies and dangerous fatigue to the body and its functional structures.

When fatigue occurs it is necessary to proportionately reduce the functional demand -or else suffer serious injury.

Could it be that the fatigue resulting in the manifestations of the body are due to the unneutralities permitted by reason of functional failure?

If it could be ascertained why, what, where and when, as influences leading to the first case of sickness in any alleged epidemic, the answer would be sufficient, —for it would have equal value in knowing the cause of each case in the series of

171

cases constituting the epidemic. It is certain that the first individual affected did not catch it from anyone else. Nor did the remainder catch it.

To illustrate the point, suppose an individual should have an acid poured or thrown upon him, along with several others. Should they, too, in being similarly affected, be thought of as catching disease from the first person injured by the acid?

Details in nature

Aside from traumatic injury, either mechanical, chemical or thermal degeneration of protoplasm is the result of deviations away from the neutral in any of these ways in which injury may occur. Such deviations would be due to functional failure or insufficiency.

General atmospheric, barometric and temperature conditions are important factors in conditioning protoplasmic irritability and thus increasing functional response. When irritability is increased, the functional response is proportionately increased. There is a corresponding use of potential energy and tendency to fatigue.

Fatigue results in slowing of fluids. Congestion follows with its inevitable train of effects. Considered together, this, of course, constitutes the condition known as inflammation. And if fluid movement is so slow as to permit degenerative processes and great enough oxygen deficiency, for too long a period of time. the cells, locally or of the entire body, will die.

State of wellness

Health is a term which implies a state of the body in which all of the trillions of living cell units comprising the human organism are normal in respect to their living processes and in functioning.

Basically, there are two equally important factors in the consideration of all human health problems, --one of which is the

172

human being, per se, and the other is the environment (both internal and external). Together, they constitute the overall responsibility of the chiropracticly educated chiropractor in maintaining a tolerable relationship between the two.

Normal health, as has been stated, depends upon adequate functional responses to every variation in the universal qualities of matter.

Variations in environmental quality are occurring in different parts of the body at all times, - but to different degrees. Considered together, without specification, all stimuli-producing conditions, substances, or combinations of such influences, are classified as unneutralities.

Stimulation is the sum total of chemical, mechanical and thermal changes in a functional cell essential to energy production in proportion to the intensity of the stimulus.

Human environment includes everything that exerts any influence upon the human body.

Stimuli arising in, or from, the environment are primary (as has been stated). All sensory nerve cells are responsive to these impulses generated. These are transmissible over nerve cell axones to their synapses with other cells, --either intermediate or terminal. A synapse is where nerve impulses from one nerve cell are transmitted to other functional cells, nerve muscular or glandular.

The number of energy units produced or released from a stimulated nerve cell body depend upon the intensity and duration of the stimulatory influence.

Health status

The subject of human health should begin with the study of the cell (which we have investigated, thoroughly).

173

The term health is quite elastic, varying in degree from perfect -or satisfactory- down to such state that living is terminated and death is a consequence.

Perfect health is experienced only when cellular environment is sufficiently neutral for the cell to make necessary adaptations without being followed by injury, as expressed in functional impairment.

The living processes in cell protoplasm constitute a continuous change in the chemistry, density, volume and temperature of the cell substance. The greater departure from normal in these qualities of the environment, the more the stimulatory influences are intensified, tending to earlier exhaustion and decrease in function.

Adequate air, food and water are the primary environmental requisites. They are obtained from fluids supplied by circulation.

In the case of body fluids, if they are toxic, they injure the cells of the entire body. Such injury is manifested by a fluid movement slow-down that results in congestion, elevated temperature and redness, --the imperative and proportionate automatic manifestations of injury.

Variations in temperature - local or general- are no different than equal variations in the atmosphere, liquids or solids. Fluctuations in body temperature depend on the rate of heat production in and dissipation from any specified area. This is not fever, regardless of duration.

Internal environment temperature, chemistry and volume are regulated by vessel wall functioning. This is primarily the walls of blood and lymph capillaries and larger vessels returnig fluid to the heart. It is at the heart, as we know, that the fluids are then, again, sent out and will reach tissues through the arterial system.

The major part of unusable chemicals that occur in the human body result from improper eating. The greater part of such poisons thereby produced are reduced by oxidation to a gaseous state and eliminated from the lungs.

The kidneys are second in importance as elimination organs. Poisons eliminated by way of the kidneys are suspended in fluids secreted by gland cells of the kidneys and expelled through the system of urinary channels. Although skin elimination is not a major factor, yet the skin is of prime importance in temperature regulation and water elimination with high external temperatures.

Environmental influences

The external environment includes everything that influences the human body --whether directly or indirectly-- from outside the body.

The threats of injury from the internal environment are quite different. These are regulated through the coordinated functioning of the nerve, muscular and secretory or glandular systems of the body.

The perpetual alternation in the constructive and destructive phases of cellular metabolism could be likened to a race between life and death in which death finally wins. In other words, we begin to die immediately after we begin to live. When the two processes are about equal, the cells are in a satisfactory state , --or healthy. But when degenerative or destructive processes are in excess of the regenerative or restorative processes, there is inevitable and proportionate sickness, with inadequate function as the major involvement.

Functional response to environmental unneutralities is the key, here. And to all who have followed this line of reasoning, it now becomes most evident.

Clarity in conjecturing

Cellular metabolism is an automatic process governed by natural law and universal innate activities within matter. Former mysteries associated with such activities have been explained away to the point that people can now depend upon the scientific conclusions that have replaced such former ignorance related to the unknown and the mysterious.

Discrediting medicine

The entire medical premise is based upon the presumption of reality in a consideration of disease entities. The disease designation is supposed to take form as a consequence of a diagnosis to establish the existence of such. But science has discredited this theory and proved diseases as entities to be nonexistent. Many scientists who do not accept the medical premise that diseases are entities believe also that alleged medications have caused more human deaths than age and all other causes. The psychological aspects of the medical premise can cause sickness mainly through fear in responding to the dour consequences of such false diagnosis.

Following misleading diagnoses, a patient is inclined to see every discomfort as due to destructiveness of the attacking disease. The patient assumes a need to use up energies to fight the disease. Such uncertainties terrify the patient to the point of increasing nerve tension and reaction, further depleting needed functional power and the sick body grows worse.

Function variation impact

Partial impairment of function causes sickness in proportion to the degree of such impairment and resulting environmental unneutrality. Complete cessation of function at any point will result in a rapid increase of the corresponding environmental unneutrality, due to retention of chemical waste from cellular metabolism and from failure to supply the amount of oxygen required for life.

Diminished oxygen supply is the most immediate cause of bodily discomfort from an increased desire for more air, --through the mildest sensation of itch to the most violent pain reaction interpreted in the centers of consciousness.

Summing up

To sum up, it can be stated that functional failure is the one condition that is responsible throughout life for all of the ups and downs in the state of health, --failure of functioning. Anything adversely affecting the body will produce unsatisfactory metabolic and functional conditions, automatically, producing characteristic manifestation --erroneously attributed to attack by some mysterious entity.

Should the body not have ability to correct the difference between itself and environment, unsatisfactory health is automatic.

A healthy body responds to environmental variations, adequately. When the body fails to functionally correct the difference between itself and its environment, then we become ill. The individual who can have the best environment is the one who will live the longest.

To be able to account for the incidence of stimuli and conditions under which the body can function in the matter of maintaining its environment is to have, at once, entry into the secrets of the human body and its life and living and the activities it produces.

Every symptom of every alleged disease is a manifestation of the body, itself, and explainable through body functioning.

Healthy regulating of the body and functioning go together.

Restoring health

One doesn't go back to restored health. Life is ongoing. We go forward. An entirely NEW status should be projected. Aim for the way it will be, --not the way it was.

GLOSSARY

Introduction

Within this concluding chapter have been included some basic considerations that apply strictly to chiropractic science. They should be examined in connection with the variations that exist between allopathic medicine and chiropractic. They are listed under their subheads with an attempt to present them with a form of continuity. They are a combination of word definitions that pertain strictly to chiropractic interpretation along with explanatory commentary. They have been organized in the form of a glossary.

New terms

In the pioneering period of scientific chiropractic there was a purposive abandoning of the medical terms of Greek and Latin derivation and a tendency to use more commonly-accepted terms to describe what was happening inside the human body and the processes involved that related to health.

There was a creation of chiropractic terms to fill the void of the medical terms that were in need of replacement.

Although Dr D D Palmer, at first, was accustomed to using the medical term disease, the term later came to be disregarded where referring to ill health. But, at first, D D Palmer made such statements as, 'Disease is too much or not enough functionating. Disease is the result of liberating too much energy, or the retarding of Innate stimulus. The former excites, the latter depresses vital force. The ordinary transformation of energy is health. The modifying, or swaying, either way, above or below normal, is disease – augmentation or lessening of impulses and morbidity of tissue.' These were the observations of D D during his early 'disease-oriented' period.

Chiropractic

Chiropractic is the overall name of related concepts advanced and considered here, in relation to their universal application to the problems of living and health, and the word will be the first considered in glossary form.

Chiropractic is the name adopted by D D Palmer in 1895. It was used to name a theory –at that time- based upon the concept that failure in the transmission of nerve energy in the human body caused every departure from the manifestations characteristic of a healthy body. Subsequent research has shown that such failure may be caused by obstructive pressure on the conduction substance or transmission elements of the nerve system (usually nerve fibers, - either axones or dendrites) .

Chiropractic deals with the laws of matter. It deals with an analyzing of matter. Through this, a practical knowledge of the subject is available.

Nothing takes place in the human body except it arises out of those factors of matter.

The explanation and description of chiropractic involvement is endless. It incorporates all that relates to the human body in sickness and health. There has been a tendency to evaluate in terms of considering chiropractic as being only the use of methods or series of acts, but such considerations disregard the important place of fundamentals that serve to establish why these acts are employed. Herein lies the crux of chiropractic.

Chiropractic is a particular and entirely different concept of human existence. It is especially related to living processes and conditions of the environment and its controls in the consideration of health. It deals with and explains every manifestation of the human body. For its best performance, it requires an understanding in the form of a blueprint that directs the chiropractic physician in employing procedures in a purposive manner.

179

The idea of neural dominance in the entire health picture especially characterizes the chiropractic concept, --therefore, the chiropractic doctor's efforts to maintain conditions of structural relations that will permit of adequate transmission of energy for appropriate functioning –the sole means by which the environment may become maintained in a satisfactory state to provide health.

The practice of chiropractic is in the application of its principles. It is limited only by the degree of understanding of its principles and the ability to apply them. Anything done for chiropractic reasons - conclusions arrived at by application of chiropractic principles- is chiropractic practice. Anything done for medical reasons is medical practice.

Life

Life, philosophically considered as a 'universal force,' falls into the scientific categorization of dealing with its nature or consistency in the form of an energy or a substance. This energy/substance, operating under favorable conditions,will induce nucleation in and of the various chemicals of non-living matter that are essential to formation of living protoplasm. And this nucleation, finally, becomes organized and classified as cells.

Life itself has seemed to be an expression of some universal principle that is manifest only for the duration of such environmental conditions in appropriate relationship.

Living is the process by which matter is conditioned for manifestations of life. And life would appear to be an automatic and imperative manifestation in certain chemical, thermal and density qualities of environmental matter, together with mysterious energy of equally automatic and imperative manifestation in living matter.

Within this instance of living, just as an overall observation, it has been found that fundamentally, moderation in life's activities can be a prime essential to the continuance of good health and extension of one's life.

Life is manifest only in an arrangement of matter. And this is primarily globular in form and designated as a cell.

Each cell is an independent unit, empowered by some principle of vital force to maintain itself in living form for a period of a hundred years or more, depending upon the ability of the body of which it is a part- to maintain a satisfactory intern al environment. This, of course, includes the understanding that there will be an avoidance of accidents arising outside the body from the external environment.

Total environment

The total environment of the human body includes everything that may exert any influence upon the human bieng. And the direct effect of environmental influence is through activity that is, in a simplified form, interpreted as either mechanical, chemical or thermal --or any combination of these factors.

The living body has rather flexible limits of tolerance for variation in such influences any of which may be of sufficient intensity to stimulate sensory cells. And these sensory cells are throughout the body. Cells should be classified as functional and non-functional. The importance of this arrangement cannot be emphasized enough.

Chiropractic vs medicine

When the fundamentals of scientific chiropractic were being explained to the public in its early days, there was always the necessity to break down the medically-accepted concept that disease was an invading enemy before explaining that chiropractic recognized what was going on, instead, as simply a disturbed condition.

The pioneer chiropractor found it necessary to deal, mainly, with the fundamentals that were involved in restructuring the body so that it would regain its proper, health functioning. The primary concern was with subluxations of the spine.

Cause

In considering basic fundamentals, the early-day chiropractor made a big issue, naturally, of 'causes and effects.' S/he explained the purpose in delivering an adjustment to the spine as being one intended to 'eliminate the cause' of ill health. But what these pioneers were really talking about were 'continuing causes.' They, sometimes, tended to overlook the need to also deal with 'original causes.' However, the differentiation became clarified as the years progressed.

Since it was explained that all functioning depended upon healthy distribution of nerve impulses through the spine, this, then, became the key to influencing health.

These were the fundamentals, as originally interpreted.

Concept

Much refinement of concept and procedures has developed during chiropractic's history, but the fundamentals related to chiropractic's basic concept continue.

Initially, evolving chiropractic was prone to make much more reference to the part played by nature than is the case, at present.

A fundamental area that was accepted as unquestionable was the reference to nature as being incapable of error. Therefore, the dependence upon natural status as a sustaining force for good.

Nerve influence

In educating the public concerning scientific aspects of chiropractic procedure, the most difficult fundamental for the public to be able to grasp in its early days was the influence of nerves upon body activity. In more recent years, there has been a more readily demonstrated understanding of this point, but to begin with, it was easy for one to connect the effect of nerve interference related to tissues in the immediate area of

182

the nerve involved, but to relate this same nerve interference to an area remotely involved was more difficult to accept.

It took years and years to demonstrate such fundamentals as commonly acceptable, today. And even now, in some instances, there is still difficulty with the concept unless intelligently explained and demonstrated.

The public has become more sophisticated than in the day when chiropractic was first presented as a science and should more readily grasp the fundamentals that serve to substantiate the procedures of the chiropractic physician.

Because of the teachings of chiropractic science, over the years, it should now be more commonly understood that there can be no organic or coordinated functioning without the transmission of nerve energy, both sensory and motor; for without both there could be no coordination of any functioning in the human body. Though this is now fairly well understood, it has been, historically, through the influence of chiropractic research that such has become more well-known and accepted.

Stimulus

The universal cause of the incidence of stimuli is the condition of matter (quality of density, chemical composition and temperature) that causes it to have that effect. It is based, first, on the tolerance of an entity for another, of the substance in one instance as to its corresponding quality in the other mass of matter. There is no stimulus without a change away from the state of the environment to which the body is accustomed, —no stimulus except under these conditions. The environment has to differ from the body before a stimulus arises.

Subluxation

The word subluxation, in order to have specific chiropractic meaning, must be in support of the discovery of D D Palmer, that obstructive pressure is caused by vertebral subluxation, only when the relation of the position of contiguous vertebrae are not, automatically, corrected by complete muscular relaxation following a return of environmental neutrality, after cessation of the stimulatory stress.

All subluxations are, primarily, protective, –if temporary. Otherwise, they exert some degree of obstruction to transmission of nerve energy and proportionately impair function of the tissues to which the impinged nerve or nerves may supply, normally, stimulatory energy impulses.

Protoplasm adaptation is the process by which subluxations become more or less fixed unless expansion of the intervertebral cartilages automatically, correct them when muscular contractions stop (either from exhaustion or because of environmental neutralization).

The elasticity of intervertebral cartilages, automatically, re-establish normal relations between approximated vertebrae in proportion to decreased muscular contraction.

Energy

Occurring in the human body is a product of the final phase of metabolism --catabolism- . It is usually --but incorrectly-- classified according to the type of cell in which it occurs, –i.e., nerve, secretory and muscular.

Of course, chemical energy and its importance to the body, should not be overlooked. But, chemical energy, properly manifested in the human body is exclusively magnetic and is responsible for the general chemical changes occurring in the living body. This is negative, not positive.

The positive energies occurring in the body are chemically produced in the process of stimulation by a stimulant which must be either mechanical, chemical or thermal. This includes all stimuli more or less comparable to the process of explosion.

184

Cells

Until a stimulus (spark) is applied to certain chemical composition, there is no kinetic energy released. These chemical compositions are formed within the functional cells of the body and - when the energy is released-- produce functional activity of the stimulated cell or cells. The energy released from a stimulated nerve cell is projected as a nerve impulse over the axone of the stimulated nerve cell (or over more or less of its axonic branches) where it serves as stimuli to other cells or gland cells to which they may be distributed. The energy released by gland cells, when receiving nerve impulses acts only upon the contractile gland cell walls, causing it to shorten, resulting in flexion or extension of joints either causing them to shorten or become narrowed, thus moving their contents.

Nerve processes extend in all directions, to and from the so-called nerve centers where the nerve cell bodies are more or less grouped, and through which the tissues of the entire body are, or may be, coordinated in their functioning. Muscular, glandular and nerve cells are the only functional cells in the body, and they are all so intimately associated by the processes of nerve cells, each of which ends in such intimate relation to a functional cell that it may deliver a stimulative impulse, thus providing for the stimulation of all functional cells in the body.

The stimuli responsible for energy release in functional cells should be classified as primary and secondary. The primary arises from the environment. The secondary arises from nerve impulses. The primary arises from the mechanical, chemical and thermal influences of the environment.

All functional cells work when stimulated, --each according to its structure. Each cell has its own peculiar magnetic quality, dependent upon the substances innately in its composition, abundantly evidenced by the particular and specific chemical composition of the different secretions of glands, i. e., mucous, thyroid, liver, pancreatic, sweat, sebaceous, lachrimal and gastric. And in a different status, but taken from the same source, --the blood and lymph.

185

Science has disclosed some special substances in the various elements characteristic of all of the different types of cells f ound in the body, but it has failed to disclose the facts which provide for the particular products of particular cells, or for the particular arrangement of the substances included and characteristically arranged in the different types of cells.

Science has not found how to create protoplasm or any of its products or by-products. Science has only learned that in certain environment, influenced by variations in chemical composition, in pressure and temperature, do cells develop into any special class, i.e., gland, muscular or nerve, and bone, ligament, cartilage, etc. However, science must admit (although that physical proof may not be available) that the first power to be considered is the inherent power derived from our ancestors.

The creative intelligence responsible for all organization of matter and energy production cannot be equalled by man in the artificialities in procedural methods supplied by science. Man has found no substitute for food, air and water, --nor can he duplicate, either. Man has found no substitution for digestion, respiration or circulation. These are the physiological activities by which the chemicals of food, water and air are processed and distributed to the cells of the entire body and from which each cell attracts the particular kind and quantity that it requires at that time, i. e., if the body is in a generally normal state.

The inherent and innate properties of the cell control the selection, quantity and use of substances brought within its immediate environment and within range of its magnetic powers.

Chemistry

General science recognizes chemistry as one branch dealing with the various substances considered under that title, making possible the recognition and classification of the elements of matter when it is disorganized, and to a very limited extent when organized.

One of the most - if not the most– distinctive discoveries in science is the fact that no chemical is a 'medicine' or 'drug' until is is so-declared by some individual or group. This is in the sense that there was no 'doctor' until the title was created.

Inflammation

The first meaning of the term inflammation relates to heat in the tissues in excess of that considered normal in a satisfactory state of health. The increased heat is the result of production at a rate above the rate of heat removal from the area and occurs simultaneously with vascular dilatation and consequent, unavoidable swelling and increased visibility of the blood in the superficial vessels, with redness increase of skin surface. Heat above the normal termperature softens the protoplasm of the cells and facilitates mechanical adaptation to the physical stresses to which the area is subjected. In case of a cut, swelling of both sides of the incision will force them together, thus closing the wound. In case of a broken bone, inflammation provides the several qualities of cellular environment to dissolve the calcium phosphate from the cells, thus softening their protoplasm until it is sufficiently molten to swell and press against each surface unit and initiate a uniting. Reossification then takes place until the bone may become even more strong than it was, originally.

Heat is normally produced in cellular metabolism and is removed by the circulatory channels. Some degree of inflammation continues in an injured area until complete correction of the injury has been accomplished. If restoration of nerve energy to vessels in the area of injury is not restored sufficiently to supply oxygen enough to keep the cells alive they will become dissolved in the fluid and form pus which, sometimes, may form in varying amounts, and if not permitted to escape through an existing outlet (opening to some surface) or, by absorption through the surfaces surrounding the cavity (pus pocket) continuing the pus, it will continue to deprive the cells in the area of oxygen and cause continued injury.

187

Inflammation is usually attributed to infection. That is a common concept and one accepted, widely. Inflammation is the inevitable effect of any injury, or any injurious influence affecting any part of the body. An individual with a generally elevated temperature is an individual who has a general inflammation. (Swelling is always an essential of inflammation. But if the whole body were to be involved, there would not be anything to swell.) The individual could have a high temperature and be sick in every other respect, but he would not have a swelling. That is the difference between general inflammation and localized inflammation. If you have the same condition in a localized portion of the body, then the fluid that gets there is not forced out by the action of the local tissues and, naturally, receiving some and not disposing of an equal amount, it increases, and we have swelling.

Whenever the fluid slows down in any part of the body, locally, or generally, so much that it does not permit the heat to reach the surface where it may escape at a proper rate, the temperature is bound to rise, on exactly the same simple basis of physical consideration as you would give to the temperature of your auto. Slowing down of fluid movement is due either to failure of production of nerve energy or failure of transmitting. If the individual is exhausted, the answer is a period of inactivity. If he is undernourished, the answer is nourishment.

Inflammation is the universal change that occurs in the tissue of the body whenever the involvuntary functions are impaired. If it is not a matter of energy production or availability, it is obstruction of transmission of energy.

Absorption

Absorption of pus by the tissues of the body is a very common occurrence. Unless it is in tissues that are not adjacent to natural cavities (such as the pleural, peritoneal or urinary), artificial removal becomes necessary. Instances are known where as much as eight pints in the pleural cavity have been absorbed and complete recovery after several years of diagnosed pulmonary tuberculosis had almost taken the life.

Circulation

Fluids are moved through lymphatic and blood-vascular systems (Functionally, they serve as one, the lymph actually being the fluid of the blood which contains organized substances constituting the corpuscles) which extend throughout the entire structures of the body. They approach all cells sufficiently close to permit them to pull –by chemical affinity– needed substances from the circulating fluids.

Congestion

Whenever and wherever the walls of blood vessels and lymph vessels of an area fail to adequately function, the movement of fluid (both into and out of the area) is reduced proportionately, except that the fluid in the weakened area is not forced out as fast as it is brought in from the unimpaired, or less impaired, adjacent area, making swelling imperative. If it is near the body surface, the superficial vessels become dilated because of the increase of their contents by reason of the difference in the rates of incoming and outgoing fluids. The incoming fluid is more than the outgoing from the area of congestion. Because of the distention of the superficial vessels, the normal color of the surface changes with an increase in redness, due to increased visibility of red blood corpuscles, --characteristic of so-called inflammation.

Changes of temperature in congested areas occur. So-called fever is merely an elevation of temperature. Heat is a continuous by-product of all metabolism in living cells, and in congested areas such heat is not removed as fast as produced. Temperature elevations in congested areas are inevitable. They are just a matter of simple physics and not dependent upon some form of disease-attack to produce such temperature elevations.

Disease

Disease is a medical term used in attempting to describe the particular sickness of a body that has allegedly been attacked by some living entity that propagates and, by diagnosis, can be

189

specifically identified. It is further contended that such diagnosis is made by observing what medicine believes to be disease-produced symptoms. Chiropractic science denies the medical concept of diseases and question the conclusions.

The human body

The human body acquires from food, air and water every ingredient required in forming saliva, tears, mucus, gastric juices, bile, the thyroid extract, pancreatic secretion and that of other glands and, in addition, forms the materials of special chemical consistency for nerve, muscle, bone, tendons, ligaments and glands, - none of which have ever been duplicated by man, in spite of the availability of science.

The human body extracts from the fluids within the body all substances unsuited to tissues and expels such through appropriate channels, thus, automatically, ridding itself of all foreign waste and unusable matter just as long as its functioning is unimpaired.

Sickness

Ill health involving the human body is inevitable when, where, if, and to the degree to which functioning is impaired. Although it is not diseases that make the body sick, when the body is sick there may be dis-ease from the slightest discomfort to extreme pain experienced. Such discomfort of pain will automatically subside in proportion to the resumption of normal functioning in the involved area or areas.

Therapy

It is not uncommon to see in chiropractic literature the reference to chiropractic as chiropractic therapy. This is sort of a careless use of language. It is not consistent with the scientific facts involved.

The word therapy carries with it the thought of the introduction of an outside force intended to arouse a force within the body to precipitate a process or result in some effect that is different than would ordinarily result.

Therapy implies a special use of some act with the thought that this will be productive of a special power that transcends the laws of ordinary powers.

To just set in motion natural laws is not a special dispensation, or therapy.

Physiology

Chiropractic science has found the word physiology more appropriate when considered in the light of work done by cells in response to stimulatory influences.

Physiological movement in the body involves the mechanics and physics of muscles.

Muscle cells are elongated and appropriately referred to as being fibers, the ends of which are attached to white connective tissue fibers which, depending upon arrangement, are either tendons or aponeuroses.

Muscle cells, when relaxed, are elongated and --when passive and not stretched-- soft and may be stretched --during which their density is gradually increased.

During contraction, all muscle cells are shortened and their transverse diameter increased, and they become increasingly firm with more violent contraction. Those attached to the skeletal structures are transversely striped and being under control of the will are classed as voluntary.

The effect of their contraction is movement of the body or some of its parts.

All voluntary muscles and muscle cells extend in a more or less straight line between their points of origin and insertion. In the latter, they are pulled toward the point of origin and involved in flexion and extension. In any event, their functioning produces either motion –if unopposed– or fixation if met by equal opposition. Science has no explanation of the details of what goes on, or how it is carried on in the contraction of muscle cells.

Nerve energy and electricity or an electric-like energy is a potentiality of nerve cells which, themselves, are like voltaic batteries in that they produce electricity by chemical decomposition or catabolism --the last phase of cellular metabolism.

As far as is known, the only different distinction between nerve cells and the cells of the general connective tissues of the body is that the nerve cells serve all functional structures by impulses reaching every functional cell in the body.

All cells produce similar energy in similar degenerative chemical processes.

All of the energy resulting from stimulation of cells of the body could be classified as electrical in nature.

Metabolism

All cells have magnetic power by which they pull into themselves all of the different substances needed for their maintenance and all purposes. The first phase in cellular activity is limited (anabolism) to securing those substances. After these are absorbed they begin to undergo change according to the kinds and quantities of chemicals in the mixture where splitting and combining of chemicals takes place and nutrients are transformed into cellular protoplasm or living matter.

In functional cells, this takes place according to how much they are required to function in ordinary and normal stresses to which the body is subjected by each individual. A portion of the food consumed is prepared and stored for cellular energy production. While the energy produced by all functional cells is similar and electric-like, they are commonly referred to as types indicating the type of cell in which the energy becomes manifest –nerve, muscle, gland–.

192

Nerve energy is a stimulus, exclusively, and if in sufficient volume, will stimulate any or all of the many cells with which the nerve cell axone (or its branches) terminate in such relation as to permit the transference of the energy impulse, projected from the nerve cell body, to enter, --whether it be nerve cell muscle cell or gland cell.

Specific activities

(A) Mental activity may involve every functional part of the body, or it may be limited to the conscious mechanism of the brain. (B) Chemical activity is a constant process in every tissue cell and in the contained fluids of the circulatory system and secretions of all glands, the air in the lungs, and in the contents of the alimentary and genito-urinary tracts. It is definitely spontaneous and occurs only within speed limits as are fixed by force of chemical affinity which attracts chemicals into and out of cellular limits, and into chemical combinations suspended in the fluids of the body. (C) Physical activity is the result of nerve, muscular and glandular functioning, conditioned by the stimulative quality or properties of the environment, and is the means whereby mechanical movement of the body through space, and the movement of all fluids act within and not a part of the cell structures of the body --is accomplished.

Nerve functioning --or generation, release and transmission of nerve energy-- could be classified as electrical production of an energy characterized by being subject to insulatory isolation and guidance, by which it is essential for coordiantion of functioning throughout the human body. And since all health is dependent, primarily, upon adequate and coordinated functioning of all functional structures, the generation, release and transmission of nerve energy is of prime importance in applying the chiropractic basic principle, i. e., nerves free from obstructive pressure.

Diet

Diet is a word of mystery, of doubtful origin and meaning. It is used to suggest that science now knows more accurately than the body when and for what it is in need in the way of food to create and maintain normal cellular protoplasm and the chemistry of the internal environment. This makes it a convenient term with which to mesmerize the laymen into securing and accepting advice of so-called dieticians.

Diet actually has exactly the same meaning as the word food, but creates more confusion and less understanding of the scientific approach to eating.

Food, when eaten by man is no more a diet than if eaten by cattle.

Hunger

Hunger is a consciousness of chemical requirements of the body, obtainable from food and by eating.

The different chemical nutrients comprising foods are subjected to the senses of taste and smell which convey to the conscious mechanism nerve impulses of such intensity that their interpretation informs as to the degree of pleasure or displeasure presented by each particular food item, thus, making it possible for future discretion in food selection.

Food and nutrition are individual problems common to all mankind from birth to termination of living, and without doubt present the highest percentage of hazards to continuing life and health.

Undigested foods

Undigested foods present the highest percentage of health hazards and living hazards to human beings. Undigested foods are as foreign to the normal body chemistry as are any of the scientifically (?) labelled drugs or medicine prescribed by those who believe in medical healing effectiveness.

Chemical irritants

Chemical irritants from improperly digested food residuals automatically stimulate, or tend to stimulate, sensory nerve

194

cells with which they come in contact and, thus, beginning the characteristic dual-directional, afferent and efferent nerve pathways of which the entire nerve system is made up and which alert the conscious mechanism of the brain. Simultaneously, or subsequently, this causes increased muscular contraction resulting in immediate heightening of the fluid pressures exerted upon the walls of all vessels or spaces containing blood, lymph or glandular secretions, also, simultaneously with the above described effects there are comparative degrees of obstructive pressure upon nerves from lessening of the size of the lumen of the intervertebral foramina in which they lie, and at which point they emit from the spinal canal.

Normally, when the body is at rest, no obstructive nerve pressure is exerted upon spinal nerves in the spinal foramina because of the characteristic resiliency of the intervertebral fibro-cartilaginous discs which, automatically, expand upon relaxation of the spinal muscles, after being compressed by violent muscular contraction in response to violent stimuli in the body, --to which the sensory nerves are unavoidably subjected.

No escape from obstructive nerve pressure is possible when there are irritants in the body, or outside, applied to sensory nerve cells. For muscular contraction (tension) is a natural and imperative result of sensory nerves being stimulated in any manner or degree, --or from any type of stimulus, be it mechanical, chemical or thermal.

Respiratory disorders

Respiratory disorders are more correctly described as conditions where excessive mucous secretions from the mucous membranes lining the nasal, pharyngeal, tracheal, bronchial and bronchiolar tubes and air sacs are present (resulting from stimulation from waste chemicals in the exhaled air). Such conditions (sustained without cessation) result in more and more degenerative changes, accompanied by characteristic inflammation (weakened blood vessel walls with dilation from failure of blood being removed as rapidly as it is carried into the area), elevated temperature and heightened sensitivity with coughing, --by which the excessive secretions are expelled from the air passages in the lungs. If degeneration is permitted to continue (by reason of malfunction), due to obstructive pressure on nerves not being intentionally removed, red corpuscles will be drawn into the congested and inflamed area in such great numbers as to have the appearance of a true hemorrhage from a ruptured wall of some blood vessel. And, in time, scar tissue will form so-called tubercles (which are only swellings in degenerative areas) followed by slow regenerative processes, just as soon as scars in any type of injury in any part of the body and not indicative of any disease entity, –but the imperative and natural manifestations resulting from obstructive pressure on certain nerves, and the resulting impairment of functioning.

Cancer

The term malignancy, as medically interpreted, strikes terror in the minds of those who accept the thought, --doctor and layman, alike. The result of this has been that the conscientious doctor, fearing delay, has just been prone to resort to radical procedures (surgical, x-ray and radium radiations) just because medicine fails in the matter of determining causative factors or successful treatment.

Medicine maintains that because of possible limited 'growth' of the malignant cells it will permit the removal of enough tissues to circumvent the entire area involved. Then, if the surrounding tissues are not already too debilitated to recover from surgery, there may be an apparent recovery. However, there is a great tendency for the condition to recur. And the average life expectancy is only a few years after surgical removal of the 'growth' and adjacent tissues.

X-ray and radiation are used on the assumption that the'cancer' cells in an area subjected to their rays will be killed without immediately killing the body cells, thus affording a respite from the ravaging processes of uninterrupted amlignancy. It is strangely paradoxical that the cell-killing and cancer-causing instrumentalities (as radiation is known to be) should be adopted as an alleged scientific means of combatting cancer.

In considering malignancy, physiologically, the theory of uncontrolled cell growth is discarded for the reason that logic, in the light of all present knowledge of cell behavior, completely fails to support it.

In the case of malignancies, medically, the approach is based upon the presumption that this is a condition in which certain cells become utterly unrestrained in dividing, --the theory of the process of cell reproduction accepted by therapy, but not accepted by non-therapeutic science.

The cause of malignancy is to be found in the common cause of tissue degeneration.

There is in the adult, tissue of an embryonic character. The diagnostician assumes these to be 'new cells.' However, a reversal of the natural cellular distribution of cellular differentiation process takes place under certain circumstances of degeneration, and it is at this stage that these particular cells are diagnosed to be cancer.

In regard to chiropractic management in cases diagnosed as cancer, it was the opinion of Dr Ratledge that there could be strong support for chiropractic effectiveness from the chiropractic ability. He maintained that the most scientific approach to the subject of human health or the health of tissues could be demonstrated by employing chiropractic procedures supported by chiropractic conclusions. And these even included tissue management in all of the alleged states and under all the names that were applied, --even cancer.

The thought, here, should not be interpreted to infer that he was encouraging the chiropractor to make claims of entering into an actual diagnosing and treating of a malfunction that had been designated under the diagnostic term, cancer; his contention was to the effect that conditions (even that referred to as cancer) are misbranded, mislabelled, and should be considered in the light of chiropractic knowledge.

Dr Ratledge was one of the few who spoke out to any extent in the matter of falsely naming degenerating tissues under the heading of 'a cancer.' And he further asserted that the science of chiropractic has succeeded in effecting the only break-through acceptable to true science as to what causes cancer. Chiropractic research has shown that there is no one cause of the condition, medically known as cancer. Chiropracticly considered, it would be found that the condition is the cumulative effect of environmental unneutralities and inadequate functioning of the tissues of the human body.

Good health is the only guarantee against cancer, –for cancer is not something that attacks. The condition is one of cell degeneration that may reach that degree from which there is no recovery. Promotion of cellular health is the only means of recovery from any degree of degeneration.

When you have a cancerous state, you have a state of paralysis in that area. The cells may be living, but that is all. And as they are just living tissue and not active, there is a natural tendency toward the retention of fluids, thus causing enlargement and also discoloration, as a structural change is taking place.

There is a general weakness of the tissues. More particular manifestations in affected tissue area follows as more tissue becomes involved as additional irritants are carried into other parts of the body.

In instances of advanced stages, where the amount of tissue involved is so great that the reactive power is low and the production of poison is so great that you will never be able to improve the environment so as to build up the cells in that area, then there should be studied consideration in terms of recommended surgery. In such cases, there is recommended a removal of the dead and devitalized cells and making it possible for the tissue cells that have sufficient vitality to react to enter the phase that is referred to as healing.

Healing is a modification of protoplasm solely by metabolism through which there is restoration of cells involved. It is regulated by the environment of the cells, themselves.

Tissue is cut and, in doing so, there is a cutting directly through some cells while in some cells there is just a little bit cut away. The factor that determines whether a cell lives is what the degree of injury has been to the nucleus of the cell.

The nucleus is the center of the cell. If the nucleus is destroyed by cutting, it dies. A chemical disturbance is produced from interference, heat is produced with an effect upon the protoplasm involved. During this process, fusion takes place and what is called healing occurs. With the gradual return of circulation, the tissue is declared to be healed.

When inactive tissue is removed, there will be tissue at the point where the injury occurs that is sufficiently vital that it can reestablish itself by its own action.

If the conditions responsible, in the first place, remain, there will be a continuous development, or redevelopment of the condition.

After surgery, patients should be adjusted to prevent the impingements that permitted the condition to develop in the first place.

Cancer degrees of tissue degeneration are caused from every type of environmental injury, --mechanical, chemical or thermal--. Every variation in any of these environmental qualities is injurious until sufficient adaptative change in the cellular protoplasm of the area establishes complete tolerance, or neutrality, at the moment.

Every injurious influence to which the body is subjected is contributory to tissue degeneration and the cancer is only an advanced degree of degeneration.

Nicotine, alcohol and all other chemicals, when present in quantities in excess, or otherwise impossible of use by the

199

body in constructive metabolism of its cells, are irritants, and, therefore, are contributory causes in degenerative processes whether to the degree of colds or cancer.

Any excessive, continued or oft-repeated, irritation from any class of irritants, i. e., mechanical, chemical or thermal, will, in time, inevitably produce the degree of cell degeneration occurring in different types and in different locations within the human body. And due to the vagaries in degree of intensity of the irritant or irritants, the period of irritation and the extent of environmental unneutrality resulting from functional impairment in the area of manifestation.

Millions of dollars are being spent, annually, in research based on a wrong theory, --that of cure--, which is unscientific. All the money in the world cannot change natural law. Our very being and maintainence of life is the product of natural law.

Everyone knows that there is a certain minimum vitality beyond which recovery is impossible. But no one knows just where that line exists.

Another factor to be considered in the cell degeneration associated with the term cancer is that inadequate nerve energy production may result from starvation of cells. Any degree of undernourisment may result from failure of proper functioning of the digestive system. At this point, it might be well to point out that all food ingested --but not digested-- becomes poisonous and definitely injurious to the tissues of the entire body, -especially affecting any weakened area that may, later, become the site of a cancerous degree of degeneration.

Is there a cancer cure? There is none. But there may be recovery. And if there is any degree of recovery, it results from restoration of the general functioning of body structures and resulting reestablishment of a satisfactory state of the environment.